THE PATIENT WILL
SEE YOU NOW

THE PATIENT
WILL SEE YOU NOW

How Advances in Science,
Medicine, and Technology
Will Lead to a Personalized
Health Care System

CAREY JAMES KRIZ

ROWMAN & LITTLEFIELD PUBLISHERS, INC.
Lanham • Boulder • New York • Toronto • Plymouth, UK

ROWMAN & LITTLEFIELD PUBLISHERS, INC.

Published in the United States of America
by Rowman & Littlefield Publishers, Inc.
A wholly owned subsidary of The Rowman & Littlefield Publishing Group, Inc.
4501 Forbes Boulevard, Suite 200, Lanham, Maryland 20706
www.rowmanlittlefield.com

Estover Road
Plymouth PL6 7PY
United Kingdom

British Library Cataloguing in Publication Information Available

Library of Congress Cataloging-in-Publication Data:

Kriz, Carey James, 1957–
 The patient will see you now : how advances in science, medicine, and technology will lead to a personalized health care system / Carey James Kriz.
  p. ; cm.
 Includes bibliographical references and index.
 ISBN-13: 978-0-7425-6204-2 (cloth : alk. paper)
 ISBN-10: 0-7425-6204-2 (cloth : alk. paper)
  1. Medical care—Forecasting. 2. Medical technology. 3. Disease management.
I. Title.
 [DNLM: 1. Delivery of Health Care. 2. Biomedical Technology. 3. Disease
Management. 4. Personal Health Services. W 84.1 K925w 2008]
 RA394.K75 2008
 362.101'12—dc22   2007044893

Printed in the United States of America

♾ ™ The paper used in this publication meets the minimum requirements of
American National Standard for Information Sciences—Permanence of Paper for
Printed Library Materials, ANSI/NISO Z39.48-1992.

In memory of my parents,
Edward and Marjory Kriz,
and Vincent O'Neill.

CONTENTS

PREFACE

SOMETHING IS WRONG with the U.S. health care system. Dramatically wrong.

In a world of exploding sciences, with the growth of knowledge on how our bodies work increasing at unprecedented levels and technologies available that are reshaping the meaning and value of all industries, the statistics on the U.S. health care system are shocking. While spending more money per capita than any other country in the world, we have *worse* outcomes on everything from life expectancy to the rates of infectious disease, at least in terms of how we compare to our global neighbors. And, along with the poor performance of our health economy, we have managed to create a system of perverse financial incentives that are paying for the wrong things at the wrong times. People in our health care industry make more money when we are sick and dying and a lot less when we stay healthy.

What are we going to do to change this dysfunctional organization of providers, facilities, and products? The answer to this question begins with a reality check on where we are in the process.

Have we constructed safeguards in society to eliminate those diseases that we know are preventable? No. According to the National Center for Health Statistics, the two leading causes of death in the United States each year are heart disease (more than 650,000) and cancer (more than 550,000). While the roots of cancer are often connected to factors that we still do not fully understand, the larger of the two—heart disease—is generally the result of lifestyle issues we do know about, with two of the largest issues being weight and inactivity. Yet we live in an increasingly obese society where our poor diets and lack of exercise border on the insane and are getting worse. Clearly, something is not working.

Are all members of society provided access to high quality care? No. The growth of the total number of Americans living without health insurance is staggering. Based on the U.S. Census Bureau's 2005 Current Population Survey our country had over 45 million uninsured living within its borders, all facing tremendous obstacles in obtaining and paying for health care services. We definitely do not have the "compassionate" society we like to advertise—at least according to over 45 million of our fellow Americans that are outside of the mainstream health industry.

Have we defined a health care community that enriches itself? Yes. The cost of maintaining the U.S. health care system is in excess of $2 trillion per year and is expected to reach over $4 trillion per year over the next decade. And who is getting this money? While it is easy and sometimes popular to target the pharmaceutical companies as the "villains" of the system, the reality is that the largest amount of expenditures—over 60 *percent*—covers the costs of hospitals and professional services. The amount spent on pharmaceuticals is only about 10 percent. We have an imbalance in our country's national expenditures, with the fastest-growing segment of our GDP in health care—consuming roughly 16 percent of our country's total budget. It is slowly killing the U.S. economy.

> Health spending is rising faster than incomes in most developed countries, which raises questions about how these countries will pay for future health care needs. The issue may be particularly acute in the United States, which not only spends much more per capita on health care than any other country, but which also has had one of the fastest growth rates in health spending among developed countries. Despite this higher level of spending, the United States does not achieve better outcomes on many important health measures.[1]

Sadly, I could easily expand the list of things that are not working in our U.S. health care system. But I also believe we are on the verge of a major revolution that has the potential to completely redefine how we think about and use health care services. Who is leading the charge? The new systems of health care will be coming from a partner that we did not even have at the beginning of the twentieth century—the computer and the evolving world of the digital.

If we mobilize around this new set of tools and the knowledge economy being defined by the genome, we could lessen (and sometimes eliminate) the impacts of disease, provide everyone in society with access to care, and ensure that all individuals have the knowledge and power to realize their human potential. And we could do it in our lifetime.

How do we start this change? The good news is that this revolution has already begun. We are lucky that some of the smartest and most dedicated members of our community are working in these emerging knowledge industries—whether looking at how to expand the power of the Internet or seeking to understand the meaning of our genome. Their dedication to discovery has provided us with the fundamental building blocks to completely transform our health care system.

We—all members of society and every level of leadership—need to get behind the power of these revolutions in thinking to dismantle and then rebuild the systems of health care we created. We should no longer be living in a world of magical ideas when it comes to health, and we should be basing our treatment plans and prevention models on real data that is validated and connected back to the individual.

What is the name of this movement? I call it *personalized health care* (PHC). Interestingly, I believe that it has its roots with one of the founding physicians of our twentieth-century medical practice, Sir William Osler (1849–1919), and his views that we need to look inside the person to understand the disease—not the reverse, which is what we have defined with our current system. To quote Osler[2], "The good physician treats the disease; the great physician treats the patient who has the disease."

ACKNOWLEDGMENTS

W RITING THIS BOOK is the result of nearly three decades of effort, starting at IBM, moving through The Johns Hopkins University School of Medicine, and finally back to industry. Along the way I have had the opportunity to engage in dialogs with a large number of people who tested my sensibilities and forced me to think of problems just a bit differently than my normal approach. So if this book has any value, and I hope that you at least find some of its ideas challenge you, it is because of this collection of individuals and the influences they have had on my thoughts—or at least my ability to integrate their ideas within my arguments.

The first person on my list to thank is Bruce Holbrook, who is probably the most unlikely individual to reference in a book like this. He is a senior partner with Goodman & Company in Norfolk, Virginia, and not the type of professional you would normally associate with the sciences and practices of medicine. Bruce has an amazing power to understand people and new ideas, and he thought it made sense for me to join a medical school and thereby introduced me to Dr. Elias Zerhouni, who was, at the time, a rising faculty member in the Johns Hopkins University School of Medicine. It was Dr. Zerhouni and Dr. William Brody, the chair of the Johns Hopkins Medicine Department of Radiology, who launched my official career in the research and clinical side of medicine and opened my eyes to its complexity and beauty. If I have achieved anything in this industry it was because Zerhouni and Brody forced me to build my own foundation and a way of approaching problems that I continue with today.

From there the journey becomes a bit more specific. My initial exposure to the fascinating elements of genetics was through Drs. Joan Richtsmeier and Craig Vander Kolk. Their combined research prowess, along with that of a number of their colleagues, exposed me to the fascinating issues of growth and how our bodies contain an almost infinite set of roadmaps.

The next major thanks I owe are to Dr. Nick Bryan, a senior member of the neuroradiology community, and my colleague on a brain-mapping project developed through an alliance of Johns Hopkins and the government of Singapore in the early 1990s. Working with Dr. Bryan and Dr. Raghu Raghavan (the director of CIeMed), I was exposed to the mysteries of neuroanatomy and the trials facing the clinical community as they worked on difficult-to-reach brain tumors.

My education and work in visualization and modeling was the product of the time that I spent with Drs. Elliot Fishman, Elliot McVeigh, and Jim Anderson. Their work and willingness to help me understand the medical challenges of imaging inspired me to think about the issues of how to best discuss health and its physical relationship to our bodies. Did we exist in dimensions and, if so, how would we express that quality in applications and on paper?

One of the most enjoyable periods of my career was the time I spent with Drs. Cathy DeAngelis, Peter Greene, Robert Replogle, Valerie Smothers, and William Baumgartner. While I was struggling with what would be the "next big thing" in medicine they demonstrated the simple and powerful elegance of CTSNet and the tremendous value of education. The end product of our discussions was the Med-Biquitous Consortium, which continues today as the hardest name to pronounce in medicine, but also one of its most important examples of a virtual community. Dr. Edward Miller was a silent partner to the CTSNet team (as the dean/CEO of the Hopkins School of Medicine) and continuously provided me with enough rope to hang myself.

Along the path of discovery in CTSNet I was introduced to Dr. Jim Fackler and his work in understanding the complexity of medicine in the intensive care unit (ICU). His observations on the problems of managing what appeared to be an unlimited number of information threads in the pediatric intensive care unit (PICU) forced me to think about this broader issue of understanding in society and how we may pushing everyone into a land of confusion. I owe Jim thanks for this insight, which I may never have stumbled upon lacking our discussions.

One of my favorite colleagues from my Minnesota period was Dr. John Kucharzyk, who is a prolific inventor and one of the most creative individuals I have met in the areas of community-based health models. Although he is better known in neuroendocrinology, John was a close friend and associate during the evolution of the team health care model I was evolving in the mid-1990s. His input and ideas were invaluable and are something I carry with me today.

I also owe thanks to Dr. Joel Saltz, who I consider one of the major innovators in the information industry. More than anyone I know, he understands the problem of medical data and is trying to solve it through increasingly clever uses of computer technology.

Beyond this group of scientists and clinicians I owe tremendous thanks to Dr. William Malarkey and the education he provided me regarding psychoneuroimmunology. This is one of the areas of discovery that I find beyond fascinating and can't wait to see where this collection of researchers moves in the future. It demonstrates the immense complexity of life and how little we understand.

Outside of health care and back to my technology roots, I have an almost unlimited number of people to thank. My various colleagues at IBM over the years, with specific thanks to Dr. Allan Scherr and Phil Joslin, are at the top of the list along with my close friend and colleague, Dave Boor. Each of these individuals dared me to be creative and push whatever talent I had into new directions.

I recently lost a colleague, Dr. Shashi Raval, who was a gifted and multitalented thinker. I tried to capture his spirit in this book, although I am sure that he would have made my job easier had he been around to read the early drafts. And on a completely different front I owe a tremendous debt of gratitude to Chris Anzalone, my editor at Rowman & Littlefield, and his publishing team. Chris waited patiently for me to finish this book and was supportive throughout, believing in the concept and the need to get the message into the world. It was a period of time not as long as building the pyramids, but it was coming close.

On the writing side I owe thanks to my contributing editor, Tami Kamin-Meyer. She reminded me of the need to maintain clarity in thought and message—and was good at ensuring that I did both.

The final collection of players I owe thanks to are my various colleagues in the business community, including Doug Hoffmeister at Accenture, Tracy Robertson at Siemens, John Dorl at Cisco Systems, and Jack Kessler of the New Albany Company. Where others may have not understood this emerging field of medicine they did, and each of these individuals demonstrated to me that it is good to have really smart people around when times are tough—and more so when they are also nice. Jack, John, Tracy, and Doug are this and more.

But finally I owe thanks to Dr. Fred Sanfilippo. Dr. Sanfilippo and I have worked together in a variety of ways over the years and it was his support and sponsorship that allowed me the time to uncover and define this field of Personalized Health Care. Dr. Sanfilippo is one of the intellectual leaders for this emerging community and clearly understands and is developing its future.

My closing thanks are to my wife, Dr. Amelia Arria, and my two sons, Alex and James, who suffered through endless discussions on how data points can go in multiple dimensions and infinitely so. If I were to put a silent dedication in this book it would be to the vast community of researchers that I have highlighted throughout this book. Their commitment to building knowledge one brick at a time will, with the proper support, change our world for the better—we need to make sure that they get our help. The next time we start looking for the real heroes of our society we should take a look in their direction.

So a big thanks to all of you mentioned above and throughout this book for helping me along the way. I was definitely able to see farther and with more clarity borrowing your vision.

PART I

THE REBIRTH OF HEALTH CARE

Medicine is a science of uncertainty and an art of probability.

—SIR WILLIAM OSLER

I N 1892, SIR WILLIAM OSLER published the first edition of the landmark, *Principles and Practice of Medicine*. Osler's book was a milestone for nineteenth-century medicine and its energized scientific foundation. Given the long and historic roots of the medical profession, it may be difficult to believe that even as recently as 1892, little was known about how to deal with the medical issues Osler chronicled in his epic work.

The dawn of the twentieth century was not a great time to contract even the most basic physical illness, like an infection, and certainly not a time to suffer from a more complicated disease, like cancer. While Osler's breakthrough book demonstrated to the medical community how to identify what ailed a patient, it exposed a new and startling reality: other than offering the seriously ill patient compassion, there was little more a doctor could do to help.

Osler's description of how physicians managed leukemia, for example, highlighted the depth of the problem: "Fresh air, good diet and abstention from mental worry and care are the important general indications."[1]

Society was beginning to comprehend the relationship of the disease process to their bodies but lacked the fundamental knowledge of how to retard those invasions. While Osler's book represented a major step forward, it highlighted what we didn't yet understand: the intricacies of how the more complex diseases can be treated. It served, in many ways, as a catalyst for discovery that began the twentieth century.

In the end, Osler's book provided the quintessential catalog of the day's mechanically focused health care industry. If a disease were to strike, it tended to follow a defined course, displaying a variety of predictable outcomes while operating within the immense complexity of the body's various interconnected systems. The tradition of rigorous science commingling with clinical practices supplemented by a strong and thorough education, promoted by Osler's work, continues to be the backbone of the medical profession.

Today, our health care communities are encountering challenges similar in impact to those confronting Osler's world. Where in Osler's time the question was whether medicine could be organized as a scientifically based profession, today we are facing a broader issue of the high costs of managing disease that could transform and eliminate the rights of all members of our society to fair and equal access to health care.

Yes, we have one of the most sophisticated systems of health care in the world—and one in which the most complicated diseases can be managed through unparalleled access to advanced technologies and outstanding professional skills. But can we continue the disparity of costs in our country's gross domestic product (GDP), in which we have grown from spending roughly 8 percent on health care in 1980 to over 16 percent by 2006? And what about the other social problems facing our society and the need to create new jobs and industries and rebuild our education system?

Each time we make an additional investment into our health care economy we need to remember that we are doing this as a trade-off to other investments our society could have made. Are we spending this money the right way? The paradox, according to an opinion survey done by the Kaiser Family Foundation,[2] is that roughly 60 percent of insured Americans are worried that their health plans are more focused on saving money than in providing good quality care. We may be spending more, but the average consumer is worried that we are not spending enough.

Given this disparity in public opinion and the reality of our health investments will we have the ability to maintain our health care system as a compassionate provider during a time of intense globalization? Unfortunately for our country, and our businesses as global competitors, while we spend 16 percent of our GDP on health care, our competitors often live in societies that spend far less than 10 percent. Without a master plan for managing our use of health resources, will the only alternative for controlling health costs be rationing? The reality is that we are probably already there—a sentiment each of us would echo every time we face a managed-care administrator telling us our upcoming doctor visit is "out of network."

And is universal health insurance the solution? If you think we have a problem today, imagine a scenario in which everyone in our county is allowed to use as much of our country's health care resources as they want, lacking knowledge of its downstream impact or how their use of health resources fits within a long-term game plan for keeping them well. While it may be hard to believe given what we know about the relationship of cigarette smoking to disease, we still have over 45 million people in the United States who smoke.[3]

The one thing I do understand is that we are not close to having a society that has a priority of making sure that each one of us understands how to build health. From the foods that we advertise in our media, to the design of our cities, we have forgotten that obtaining health is not simply showing up in a clinic when you feel ill. It is a journey and a series of decisions that we each make each day and, unfortunately, often do so given a context of clouded messages on what is good and not good for us.

The next time you get into our car to drive to the mall or walk down the aisles of the local grocery store, are you aware of the choices you have made that day or are about to make and their impact on your body and your health? The data[4]—*over 60 percent of Americans are either overweight or obese*—suggests the answer would be no.

We have a messy collection of intertwined problems to solve.

Although not intended as the definitive answer to every question facing our health care system, *The Patient Will See You Now* will address the evolving landscape of medicine while proposing a major transformation on what it means to be healthy and live—and at least start the discussion on how to rebuild our industry.

One thing that is abundantly clear: the issues confronting our health care system can be resolved only by a diversity of ideas. While managed and rationed care are interesting social experiments, for example, they fail to address the more pressing need to remold the health care system into one in which economic incentives are aligned, consumers are aware of their choices, and each of us works with a team of professionals—not simply a physician or a cost-focused insurance company—to define, control, and build health.

Finally, given the complexity of the questions and answers facing our health care system there is little doubt that society has moved beyond the era of the isolated and solitary scientist, researcher, or physician curing the ills that plague us. The coming effort required to redefine and reposition our health care system calls for an unprecedented course of action and cooperation from everyone—whether they are a member of the medical community, the information industry, or a patient.

Something is about to change and there is no doubt it will be dramatic.

Health Care in the Twenty-First Century

In Osler's day, having strep throat—to provide one example—was a potentially life-threatening event. Today, society generally accepts a number of truths about health and illness. Among the most basic is the notion that infections can be treated through antibiotics. This may not sound like a major accomplishment, but our nineteenth-century relatives would likely have been astonished that an infection could be treated by a simple pill.

By the end of the twentieth century a host of "miracle" drugs were invented to combat a variety of illnesses, with the discovery of antibiotics being one of the most revolutionary. Fortunately, mankind's medical ingenuity did not stop there. It extended beyond pharmaceuticals to discover new ways of surgically correcting problems that otherwise could have spelled an instant death sentence. Whether dealing with conditions of the heart or searching for novel approaches to eliminating cancers, society is immersed in a period of intense innovation that has resulted in a flurry of new approaches to managing disease and improving the quality of life.

In the end, man's inventiveness has provided society with an increased understanding of how the human body functions and responds to its environments. With the potential for establishing optimal health—not simply disease management—as the lofty goal for all members of society, this innovation and motivation is a far cry from where society was one hundred years back, yet it is only a limited introduction of where medicine could be by the end of the next one hundred years.

We have become experts on the mechanical activities of our bodies. So where do we go from here?

Welcome to a world of uncertainty.

Entering the Unknown

The Patient Will See You Now explores both the general and mechanical view of health while introducing the emerging concept of personalized health care (PHC). The practices and systems of PHC are ushering in an era of change Osler would no doubt have both appreciated and defended as a natural progression in the scientific methods he espoused in his epic work.

A question Osler subtly raised that is demanding more attention in today's technologically advanced world is how does medicine peer inside the individual to understand the disease?

There are actually two schools of thought that respond to this inquiry. One method is mechanical and defines the state-of-the-body-as-a-machine as it exists in a single moment in time. The other is time based. It provides a series of paths that predict the body's destiny, with an obvious correlation to our genes, the complex engine of our growth and inheritance housed within each of our cells.

However, the story of PHC involves more than merely comparing a collection of genes and mechanical systems. It focuses on how these genes are defined, how they evolve and react to the environment around them, and, finally, how they regulate man's ability to enjoy the world. It is a complex tale that society is only just beginning to understand.

When we can finally decode the script of our lives housed in our genome, it should prove a compelling read.

Core Values of Personalized Health Care

Scientists assume, although with a strong degree of certainty, that the human body is regulated by its DNA. Moreover, scientists understand this regulation involves an array of complicated factors and raises some complex questions. How does this emerging knowledge of the genome, chemistry, and biology impact life? The answer begins with a few observations and "truths."

Truth 1: The human body is composed of complex systems that govern health and disease.

Every moment of our lives is composed of a mixture of actions and behaviors we consciously govern and those our brains manage for us. These activities of living are regulated by various bodily systems controlled by a complex interplay of actions governing every aspect of our lives, from communications to nourishment to waste management and cellular repair. Fortunately, the brain has evolved into the world's most sophisticated thinking machine with the ability to manage these system controls for us—and largely without our direct oversight. Imagine, for example, how difficult life would be if we had to worry each second about how to feed and fix the trillions of cells contained in our bodies.

Truth 2: The human body has adaptive strengths.

Among the most amazing characteristics of the human body is its ability to adapt to complex and changing environments. For example, when the body senses something remiss in its surrounding environment, it automatically engages in a series of covert events designed to make it easier for you to respond. This "fight or flight" reaction—the near instantaneous increase in our body's levels of adrenalin and cortisol that causes our heart rate to speed and increases the blood flow to our major muscle groups—is the ultimate case study in how quickly the human body can supercharge itself in exigent circumstances.

Truth 3: All bodies will age and die.

Is the aging process inevitable? Do humans have the ability to retard the impacts of time and reverse the slowly cascading decay it introduces? The questions of cellular reproduction and how our bodies mature and eventually die is one of today's more captivating research issues. Society's future systems of PHC will begin framing this important issue with piece-by-piece breakdowns of how the body appears to live through a series of programmed events while following some form of internal destiny.

Through increased knowledge of this *mission*-oriented growth, will mankind ever have the power to unwind the inevitable pairing of birth with death?

Book Organization

The chapters of *The Patient Will See You Now* will navigate through a number of technical concepts that I believe are staging the transformation of the industry while remaining true to a basic premise: science is largely operating within a world of unknowns and there will be no easy fixes.

I do not believe, for example, that the answers to the questions facing us today about access to and the costs of health care will be found by simply providing everyone with enough money to cover the costs of health insurance or even to make that insurance portable. Nor will the difficulties be solved simply by building more hospitals or graduating more physicians, nurses, and additional health care providers.

Why not address the more fundamental questions? Rather than throwing more resources at our current health care systems, I urge society to reevaluate the root causes of the health care crisis of escalating costs, worsening health statistics (as compared to other developed countries), and finally the problems of the uninsured by shifting the issues back to the core questions of living and destiny. The ultimate goal of this realignment of attitudes should be for every person to understand and actively participate in his or her own unique personal health mission.

Guess what? That exact type of health care system was alive in our society before the twentieth century and our explosion of new ideas. Unfortunately our technology-driven way of life in the twenty-first century, while providing a wealth of new opportunities, has also blinded us to the intense human elements of living. We are becoming more isolated, dependent on complex systems for basic survival, and have destroyed some of the most basic forms of social support.

Is e-mail, for example, the best way for us to communicate? And didn't the recent Katrina disaster show us how incredibly fragile our world can be?

Why not allow each of us to take control of our health with the right tools at our disposal: outstanding science, medical guidance, and real options that address our unique biological potential as our supporters this time? And the pieces of this puzzle are already staring at us waiting to be assembled into a coherent and meaningful picture. The ultimate irony is that our movement back to the past of a human-engaged health care system will be driven through an environment of complex technologies that we introduced in the latter half of the twentieth century and have continued to nurture in the twenty-first and many today view as having dehumanized us in the first place. It's no wonder we are often confused: our world is filled with paradoxes.

The Patient Will See You Now is divided into four parts covering various elements of the PHC solution. Part I contains the broad and guiding principles of this new form of health care. Part II explores the complexity of our expanding world of information and how with each additional discovery we seem to uncover an increasing array of more complex problems. Part III will dive into the enabling technologies that are helping us manage and redefine heath and represent a co-revolution of invention spanning the microprocessor to the Internet. The projected impact of these converging threads will be woven together into the final section, part IV, which discusses the evolution of the health care system to the impending rise of the empowered consumer. Here we see what the future could plausibly mean for you as a health care consumer.

It is my hope that by this book's final chapter, you will find the choreography of genetics and the information revolution that will define our systems of PHC important and captivating. It will be an interesting century.

Notes

1. Sir William Osler, *Principles and Practice of Medicine*, 1892.

2. "Kaiser Public Opinion Spotlight," Kaiser Family Foundation, January 2006.

3. "Decline in Adult Smoking Rates Stall," Centers for Disease Control, October 2006.

4. "F is in Fat: How Obesity Policies are Failing in America," Trust for America's Health, 2007.

CHAPTER 1

THE BODY AS A MECHANICAL SYSTEM

WHETHER YOU BELIEVE that we—that is, *Homo sapiens*—have evolved from some lower-order species à la Darwin or are the product of a master plan through creationism, you will nonetheless accept a number of core tenets of "being." All of us know, for example, that we need to consume food for energy, that we need to breath, and that our bodies require sleep. While we may not understand how all of the biological systems of our bodies connect or how they acquired their function in the first place (e.g., the way the heart works with the circulatory system), we have through our actions at least demonstrated a tacit acceptance of the most basic principles of life. Our bodies are machines and we generally understand that they have certain survival requirements. And although we may not manage our survival requirements as well as we should, we are at least trying—and our systems of health care have been there to help us along.

You can easily argue that the theories of our body's *mechanics* have laid the foundation for our health care system since the birth of the science of medicine—with the knowledge that errors will appear, serving as the basis for disease. Fortunately, medicine's efforts to manage and control many of these mechanical problems have proven successful. For example, medicine has invented ways of beating back infections, repairing broken parts, and even retarding the ravaging impacts of aging. Medical researchers have even learned how to control the more abstract problems of disorders like diabetes, where the body's systems fail to provide the correct mixture of chemicals to sustain the body's conversion of glucose to energy.

The tragic story of the late Christopher Reeve highlights just how important and fragile these system components of our body can be—and how complex their relationships can be among themselves.

On October 11, 2004, Christopher Reeve died from complications of a systemic infection. His death that Sunday afternoon marked the end a journey that had begun in Culpepper, Virginia, on May 27, 1995, less than a decade earlier.

On that fateful spring day, Reeve, an avid equestrian and accomplished actor, fell from his horse, severely fracturing the C1–C2 vertebrae of his spinal cord, two of the most important and fragile connections of our body. The average adult spine consists of twenty-six vertebrae, with C1 being at the very top—and the last in line as the spinal cord enters the brain. The resulting trauma of Reeve's now fractured C1–C2 vertebrae rendered him paralyzed from the neck down, unable to breathe on his own or move his arms or legs. While Reeve was fortunate to have survived the fall, the mishap introduced sweeping changes to his body and was the start of what became a cascading array of mechanical breakdowns.

The reality is that our bodies are built with a network of systems; some are obviously interrelated while others are only tangentially linked. The classic systems include the *circulatory, digestive, endocrine, immune, lymphatic, muscular, nervous, reproductive, respiratory, skeletal,* and finally the *urinary system.* Are there more systems to discuss? Clearly our bodies can be characterized through a number of interactions, from these higher-level activities to the small systems operating within an individual cell. The point is that our bodies can be defined by a number of organized "systems" spanning the depths of our cells to the gross anatomy of our bodies—and with mechanical features and chemical properties that operate within an incredible set of balance and control.

Unfortunately in Christopher Reeve's case, his riding accident disrupted one of the most fundamental support structures of the body's mechanics—the central nervous system and its vast network of connections that support everything from breathing to the feeling in our toes. In less than one clock tick, Reeve had destroyed a highly tuned example of the elegance and intelligence of the human body.

Think for a moment of the architecture of the spine and how it is designed to protect this critical neural structure. The nerves that build your spinal cord are among the most sensitive linkages in the human body. Along with protection, the surrounding vertebrae provide dual values as they maintain the body's form and structure. And these vertebrae do their job with a maximum of flexibility and power—allowing our bodies to twist, turn, and still maintain the integrity of the spine's vital inner layer, while they manage the literally billions of instructions moving around the body to the brain. It is a task of immense complexity and mystery.

Imagine the mess you would have if you were trying to eat a meal and it took five minutes for your body to react to the required movement of spearing through a salad, then waiting again to lift your fork to your mouth. Don't forget chewing and swallowing. Now try coordinating a knife and fork as you try to cut your meat. These tasks are made simple and are efficiently managed by the brain through a well-planned conduit of nerves traveling from the brain through the spinal cord to a seemingly endless number of neural connections.

The good news is that the spinal cord is also one of the countless examples of superior engineering and fail-safe design. The process of connecting the desired actions of your brain to the peripheral nerves controlling the functions of your hands and fingers works well and generally can take care of and repair many problems. At least it does in most cases.

Christopher Reeve's accident is an example of a system issue his body could not repair. The connection between his brain and certain peripheral areas of his body had been severed, forcing a cascade or domino effect of system failures.

While just one of the numerous systems of the body, the nervous system plays an integral role in almost all life functions. Although it could be argued that other more dramatic systems, such as the heart and lungs, are at least equally as important, there is no doubt the body's need for the information conduits contained in the nervous system renders it of unique value. On another level, it is also an excellent example of how the body operates through a connection of systems, with the downfall of one potentially impacting the health of another.

Mechanical Breakage

On the surface, spinal injuries are an easy-to-understand set of actions and reactions. The brain, operating on a set of data points and our own limited abilities to understand our environment, helps guide the movement of systems. The toes, for example, contain both sensory neurons (those that inform whether you stepped into hot water) and control (those allowing you to move your toes from the hot water to dry ground).

The ultimate beauty of our bodies is how effortlessly these unique systems are unified within a carefully orchestrated series of actions and reactions. And some of our more complex systems operate without our having any conscious awareness of how they work—or why they do so. The heart pumps, the immune system reacts, and the stomach digests, all through the complex control of the brain and some blueprint operating largely outside of our understanding.

What happens when these systems begin to malfunction? Why does the immune system, in some cases, turn on the body, inflicting damage on other internal systems? For anyone with multiple sclerosis (MS), this facet of system reactions has a script that seems to follow its own predestined set of pathways. Because for those with MS the body acts, but in a way that is both damaging and potentially deadly—there is an internal error in the body's control.

The concept of evolution within a disease pathway is an example of how the *mission* elements of our bodies impact these more fundamental *mechanical* systems. Let's say, for example, a tumor of a certain size is growing silently within your body. It is only when the tumor reaches a specific critical mass that its size and spread begin to disrupt the life-sustaining systems of your body. Prior to this evolutionary stage, the tumor coexisted peacefully with you.

We also know that *mechanical* systems break. If you own a car, you have no doubt experienced the frustration of having a car part malfunction. Your brakes wear out, the engine may not turn over, or a tire goes flat. These experiences are part of life and teach us that mechanical things are susceptible to breakage.

What causes these operating failures? There are a number of issues, ranging from breakage caused by accidents, to flaws in physiology, to invasions by bacteria or infection. Yet, considering how little we understand its root causes, the scariest of these error agents tends to be cancer, the ultimate uncontrolled freeloader.

On one level, cancer is not that complicated.

Yes, it can cause massive amounts of medical problems and complications, even death. Anyone afflicted with cancer understands the fear of having it invade their bodies. Facing the untold damages it can wreak upon the body's systems along with undergoing repeated treatments and taking medications are experiences only a fellow cancer patient or survivor can relate to.

It also represents the ultimate example of the unknown power of life—we are not sure where cancer comes from and why it strikes. But on another level, cancer is "simply" a collection of cells that are not part of the body's master plan that cause interference to the programmed functions of the body. It is when these cancer cells leave their initial home to invade and otherwise disrupt the programmed activities of their neighbors that medical problems ensue.

The reality is that cancer cells also have little to do other than feeding themselves and growing. They act in isolation from the rest of the body's choreography, figuring out ways to reproduce and steal nourishment while adding little value beyond their selfish ability to procreate.

Now compare cancer cells to those cells designed to control the body's *mechanics*, which must somehow develop ways of working together within the body's larger "system" model. Your lungs have a job to do in capturing oxygen and propelling it through the blood stream to feed the body's literally trillions of endpoints, which they somehow understand as part of the body's larger design. When cancer cells invade, preventing the various components of the lungs from accomplishing their primary task, the result is devastating for the systems your lungs support. It can also lead to death.

While the amount of coordination occurring at a body's cellular level represents one of the more fascinating points of our evolution, these *mechanical* elements are generally easy to understand, at least at a conceptual level. It is common knowledge, for example, that people need a certain amount of sleep per night and that we need to consume food and water to survive. It is also common knowledge that certain actions or behaviors can cause devastating impacts on our health, sometimes leading to premature death.

Putting aside the issue of why things go wrong in the first place, society has managed to develop a number of creative solutions to various medical maladies, with some of the more important mechanical fixes including heart bypass and knee replacement surgeries, pacemakers, glucose monitors, and chemotherapies. Figure 1.1, which contrasts the thinking of a *mission* and *mechanical* focus in health care, highlights the overarching themes in *mechanical* corrections (the "what" question)—and our ability to identify the corrupted system and component and then define a replacement that will work in concert with the body's systems, whether caused by disease or trauma. The more subtle, but equally important, issues of our bodies are governed by its *mission* (the "why" question)—and the impacts of aging and design on both disease and health states.

In the end, humans are a living organism housing a large number of independent systems working together and equipped with powerful ways of both protecting themselves from intruders and oftentimes repairing themselves. But unfortunately someone failed to give us a maintenance manual to explain its complexities or how to improve its performance.

Your car mechanic works under completely opposite conditions and has the luxury of being able to reference an exhaustive amount of information on the inner workings of your vehicle to help determine what will be required to fix an observed problem. You may not

Figure 1.1. Mission and Mechanical Focus in Health Care

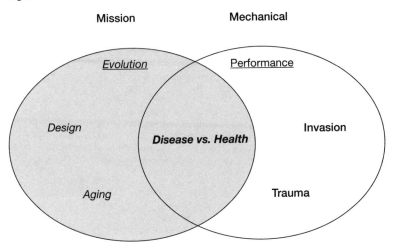

like the mechanic's diagnosis or how much it will cost you to repair the car, but if the mechanic is trustworthy, he at least gave you a description of what's wrong with the car along with a solution grounded in a solid foundation of facts.

Wouldn't it be incredible if it was that simple to diagnose what ails the body? Luckily for us sometimes our bodies have the ability to correct problems on their own.

A Self-Healing World

A curious phenomenon of life is that the various systems of our bodies tend to reinvent themselves when confronted by changing environments. A case in point is the physiological change of populations living in mountainous cultures.

Were you to spend the next year living in an elevated atmosphere, you would notice some changes in your body and lungs as they adapt to what they recognize as new requirements for your mechanical structure. A lung is, in simple terms, a mechanical device that captures volumes of air within a number of internal sacs of tissue. Repeating its breathing exercise with the oversight of your brain, the lungs begin adapting to the change in environment by enlarging their overall size. This occurs to accommodate the need to acquire larger volumes of air to accomplish the same job the lungs performed when you were living in a lower-level atmosphere and a less dense concentration of oxygen.

The lung is operating under the basic premise of a self-healing machine that reads and adjusts to its changing world, ensuring that its job still gets done while it adapts—although this occurs only up to a point and, in some cases, for only so long. Dramatic trauma, like the type introduced by lung cancer, for example, is one of those cases where the lung is not normally able to self-correct an error in its internal operations.

Unfortunately for Christopher Reeve (and us), the spinal cord is an example of a major system that is not that malleable—the nerves of the spinal cord do not typically regenerate, or at least they will not do so on their own. So an error here, whether introduced by disease or trauma, will often have devastating consequences.

But the spinal cord is not alone. There are other diseases of omission or error in which the body cannot maintain its natural balance without outside help.

I should know. I have one of those devastating diseases: I am a diabetic.

Like others so afflicted, I have a problem in my pancreas and in the way my body deals with and manages insulin, the hormone created and regulated by the pancreas that helps to control the body's glucose levels. My body does not produce enough insulin to keep me alive, and without man-made intervention I would be dead.

I am a walking miracle of our human invention and subsequent intervention and live because scientists know enough about how the various systems of my body operate. They have devised a clever way of augmenting my body to help fix the system error I have within my pancreas. I represent, as do my fellow diabetics, a success story for science in which my individual system failure does not lead to a general system breakdown. While not a perfect solution, I live with this fix and enjoy a more or less normal life.

Unfortunately, Christopher Reeve did not have the luxury of options I was offered. Facing a problem of multiple dimensions (the inability of this particular cell to regenerate, the loss of the information conduit, the impact on downstream systems), his individual system failure was beyond the fix options of current science and will await discoveries in areas ranging from signal management to cell regeneration. And while I have not been cured (I simply manage the consequences of my system failure), I am nonetheless able to continue living and avoid the larger general breakdown and death that Christopher Reeve experienced.

Reeve was, in the end, a victim of our lack of knowledge and the reality that his body was facing a problem beyond its corrective powers. And although his medical errors have been easier to understand than mine, they were far more complicated to repair on a biological level. While my body reacts well to foreign-made insulin, Reeve's body accepted only his native neural cells and their connections housed within his spinal cord.

So where will our research on *mechanical* issues move in the future? I believe that this new generation of discovery will be based on, among other things, a greater appreciation for the *mission* elements of our bodies—or our increased understanding of how our bodies evolve and mature over time. Other forms of discovery will come through the growth of innovative ways of including man-made devices within our bodies to either replace or augment failing components. Some of the more interesting have been in the growth of the implant industry for replacing aging bones (knees or hips, for example) and the various attempts to model and replace the mechanics of the heart.

A larger question is in what defines and oversees these *mechanical* systems. Our genome is the script, but what mediates its various genetic markers—and how can we influence them in the future? Are cancer and heart disease avoidable? Why couldn't science figure out ways to fix the nerve breakages experienced by Christopher Reeve in his riding accident?

Welcome to several of the problem sets of *mission*-driven health care.

CHAPTER 2

MISSION AND THE EQUATION OF LIFE

O N JUNE 15, 2005, Dana Reeve, the wife of the late Christopher Reeve, was diagnosed with an aggressive, and what would later emerge as an incurable, form of lung cancer. It was an unspeakable second tragedy to the Reeve family and their surviving young son.

Why did this happen? Unfortunately, Mrs. Reeve's medical history contained no obvious explanations as to why she was included in the world's escalating number of lung cancer victims. Moreover, traditional cause-and-effect relationships did not provide much insight.

No, Dana Reeve was not a career smoker.

A large percentage of lung cancers are caused by cigarette smoking, and typically in those with a rather extensive smoking history, but the usual correlation between smoking and lung cancer did not apply to Dana Reeve. From what was known about Mrs. Reeve, she was a nonsmoker and did not come to her doctor's office after a twenty-year history of smoking a pack a day.

She was also not a factory worker exposed to an array of the obvious cancer-causing agents.

The next most likely causes of lung cancer are the carcinogenic chemicals found in the modern and emerging industrial world, including asbestos. While no one can be absolutely certain what she might have been exposed to, her career in acting and modeling did not match the profile of the average factory worker.

Lastly, Mrs. Reeve was not a descendent of a family history loaded with cancer survivors and victims.

Sometimes, and this is based on the imperfect world of statistical analysis, cancers tend to cluster in families and within communities of related parties. Mrs. Reeve apparently had a relatively normal set of genetic trees, with no obvious "smoking gun" in her family that would have pointed to this unfortunate diagnosis.

So what caused her death? She died based on a *mechanical* dispute—forcing one of the many systems of her body into a failure state, eventually causing a larger and pervasive system error and, eventually, death. It is sad to say, but Mrs. Reeve was simply one of the more than 150,000 lung cancer casualties that have occurred each year since 1995[1]. Although Dana's and her husband's deaths were the end products of very different root causes, their deaths shared a common bond: both were the result of breakdowns in how the various connected systems of their bodies worked.

However, Mrs. Reeve's death exemplified an even more powerful concept: the broader question of *mission*. This involves asking how the cancer that grew within her body started in the first place before deciding to expand and then eventually invading enough of her normal systems to wrest away control and eventually take her life.

Where do we find the answer to these mind-numbing questions—why Dana Reeve and why then? To gain an understanding or starting point for these questions, we must step back and discuss a number of key concepts unrelated to the physical cancer housed within Mrs. Reeve's body. The first is the concept of time.

Living with Time

People who have visited the Grand Canyon have, even unconsciously, grappled with this dilemma. The life span of a human is brief, if measured in geologic time. Think of it this way: the average life expectancy for someone living in the United States is approximately seventy-eight years old. By comparison, the average life span of a fruit fly is about two weeks.

Although there are other creatures on this earth whose average life spans are longer than humans (including some turtles and trees), organic life generally has a well-defined glide ratio to its end state. You will not find too many people who live past one hundred years, for example, and no one has lived to age two hundred. Not too many dogs live past age thirty, either.

The Grand Canyon epitomizes just how short a period of time seventy-eight years really is—and why it is important to begin appreciating the finality of our bodies in this physical dimension of our world.

It is estimated that it took almost 2 billion years of geological forces to define the expanse and depth of the Grand Canyon. The various continental shifts and erosions took an extremely slow yet deliberate toll on the geology of the Colorado River, with the Grand Canyon representing one of the world's most stunning examples of geologic evolution. If you were to judge these changes during any seventy-eight-year period, chances are any differences you might notice would be negligible.

To understand the mission elements of your life, first accept the basic premise that you are living in a finite body with a particular number of years to live and that your body will be subject to a variety of forces that impact how well you react to time and the variables of life. And many of the long-term changes you will eventually notice in your body, appearance, hair, skin and the like are due to forces that ebbed and flowed during your short life span—and may have gone generally unnoticed.

The majesty of the Grand Canyon is clearly stunning when viewed today. But as you look down to the canyon's floor, or watch the water weave through its beds, are the reasons the canyon took its grand shape obvious?

The answer is probably no, and for good reason. People tend to live moment-to-moment, with little future thinking or appreciation for how individual and subtle changes may be taking place within our bodies—or how the forces of nature are continuing to change the Grand Canyon.

The challenge each of us faces is how the countless decisions we make every day will impact the *mechanical* state of our body in the future. Do our behaviors enhance either our optimal health status or life span? Understanding the concept of evolution over time as well as how things can and will change based on a life script and environment are key elements to appreciating one's own physical characteristics and limitations.

Relating this analogy to the spread of Dana Reeve's cancer, at what point in time did that first renegade cell that eventually figured out how to replicate, grow, and invade her lungs first appear? When, in the timeline of her life, did some perhaps arbitrary collection of data points conspire to change, turning what was once normal and customary inside her body into a seed for a complex killer?

The place to begin the journey is by looking in the mirror.

Knowing Who You Are

Almost every time you begin a physical exam or show up in a clinic for treatment of an illness, a member of the medical staff will ask you questions about your life. Standard inquiries include a brief family history and the symptoms of your illness. This set of small data points provides your healthcare providers with insight into what you may be predisposed to. For example, a family history of cancers may make you a more likely candidate yourself, along with offering obvious clues of some later diagnosis.

For another example of mission-based thinking, think of the typical high school reunion: why did some of your classmates look better than they did twenty years ago and some worse? Some aged more than others, some died, and almost everyone generally appeared as only a hint of the physical person you once knew.

The answer to this question begins with the same fundamentals your health professionals were trying to decipher when they asked you questions about your family history. They were trying to grasp the more obvious clues to what could be contained within that internal roadmap of your body otherwise known as the genome.

We will explore the broader meaning of the genome and its relationship to the future of medicine later, but for now let's work with a basic description: the genome contains the potential scripts of how your physical life could unfold. It is critical to recognize the disclaiming word of "potential," because one aspect of the genome is clear: much of the future impacts of the genome will involve a number of complex interactions within your body that unfold over time and could vary based on an unknown combination of events.

The causes of those interactions are one of the major discoveries and foundations for the emerging sciences of personalized health care (PHC).

Scientists generally assume that a number of human genome components were set at birth and are not subject to much variation. For example, more than likely, you were born with a projected eye and hair color and will reach a certain physical height with a predestined body type. Many of these more mundane physical elements appear to be preprogrammed factors we each simply have and cannot change—at least without some form of genetic engineering.

Now, consider the errors in our *mechanical* systems that cause death or reduce our abilities to enjoy our surrounding environment—with lung cancer as a way of starting the discovery. Why do some of us get cancer and others do not?

Dana Reeve, for example, seemed to have done everything right yet she still came down with it. Moreover, almost immediately after her diagnosis, she died. Did something in her environment cause the cancer? Or did she have a genetic marker that no one was able to understand?

The answers to these questions raise a large number of issues of data collection and correlation, with the objective being to establish the causal relationship between some event (or events) in Dana Reeve's life and her eventual disease condition. Fortunately, a number of other examples of environmental influences on health and disease are more obvious. The residents of a small town outside of Buffalo, New York, provide an unfortunate example of how the supposed safe haven of your home can become a toxic and deadly environment.

The town, Niagara Falls, is known more for its famous waterfall than its surrounding neighborhoods—and especially not the neighborhood located on a small parcel of land called Love Canal. Hopefully, the sad legacy of this story will never again be repeated.

Love Canal and Our Life Script

The industrial age of the United States was a time of tremendous wealth and economic growth for our young country. The world was rapidly shifting to systems of organized production with many of the coastal (and riverfront) towns becoming the centers of early industrial activity.

Western New York was one of the areas in the United States that benefited from this changing world of business, with Love Canal simply representing yet another sliver of the many middle-class homes in a neighborhood near the Niagara River.

Unfortunately, however, Love Canal suffered from a huge problem. Within the confines of this fifteen-acre plot of land 42 million pounds of toxic chemicals, including PCBs, were buried underground, placed there by the Hooker Chemical Company between 1942 and 1953. PCBs have obvious linkages to disease in humans, but the unsuspecting mothers, fathers, and children of the Love Canal neighborhoods continued living atop a toxic dump of potentially lethal chemicals generated by Hooker Chemical.

As with most changes that occur over time, the people of Love Canal lived quietly, although you can safely assume that many wondered about the annoying stench that seemed to permeate their small community. Unfortunately, this odor also represented one of the classic examples of a disease-fostering agent—and a chemical that would eventually modify a number of the core body systems and introduce potentially life-threatening changes. Unbeknown to them, the residents of Love Canal were coexisting with an extremely dangerous collection of *life equation* variables.

Love Canal is one of the most blatant examples of the potential there is to alter the preprogrammed missions of our body. PCBs and the other toxic chemicals housed within the Love Canal dumping ground defined and accelerated the disease processes in people that would have more than likely had a very different script written within their genome.

Whether or not they liked it, or even realized what they were doing, the residents of Love Canal were demonstrating the power of an individual's actions and their environment to define a new evolutionary path for their bodies. The change for the residents of this victimized neighborhood included a number of new and unexpected endpoints spanning cancers, various disfiguring illnesses, and even early deaths. And sadly, their exposure to the toxic soup beneath their otherwise quaint streets provided a rewrite to their later chapters that was both unfortunate and unnecessary.

Something important to remember is that while mission thinking provides a rich collection of long-term problems to solve, they must also be put in a context of their relationship to the *mechanical* systems of our bodies. As living and dynamic organisms, it is critical that we appreciate both the general and specific ways the many systems of our bodies unite, how they evolve over time, and how they change and adapt to the many disruptive forces that cross their path.

As anyone involved in the discovery of new pharmaceuticals (like Vioxx, for example) can tell you, figuring out how to precisely connect an action with the complex and sophisticated systems of the body is no easy task. How can researchers know for sure when they build their case for a new discovery that impacts one of the body's many systems that it will work for absolutely everyone in an even, predictable manner?

The answer is they can't, at least given today's knowledge. And, as the tragedies associated with Vioxx and the Love Canal demonstrate, that absence of predictability can be devastating.

Still, there is also a clear difference between the two scenarios. In Love Canal a number of known variables that directly impacted the health of neighborhood residents were introduced that resulted in almost universal changes for everyone and without their knowledge.

Vioxx acted differently within different people (the "Vioxx Impact"), all of whom had knowingly taken the drug.

So what is the connection between lung cancer, Love Canal, and Vioxx?

Lung cancer is a nasty disorder often linked to some behavior or environmental force. It is, given our current knowledge base, an almost always fatal condition that usually appears with little warning. Many people with the disease today may simply complain of a chronic cough while continuing to keep up the paces of their busy lives, such as working, enjoying friends, or playing sports, all while not displaying signs of its presence.

However, a few relatively well-known relationships link certain behaviors with the incidence of lung cancer. If you smoke, your odds of contracting it dramatically increase. If your family history is filled with victims of cancer, you have a much higher set of odds. Finally, if you have been exposed to a number of known carcinogenic—cancer causing—chemicals, the likelihood of getting cancer increases, too.

But does having these sets of environment variables or a family history guarantee you will get lung cancer? No, they don't, and it is exactly this type of uncertainty and unpredictability that makes medicine so messy today. Such was the case for Dana Reeve. Contracting cancer is not as simple as adding 1 + 1 to get 2.

Life Equation: H = F(A, G, E)

Math and statistics, while sometimes difficult-to-understand sciences, can be extremely useful in defining and managing the complexities of our lives. Knowing that water freezes at 32 degrees Fahrenheit is, for example, an important law of our physical world allowing us to conclude with some certainty that if the outside air temperature is twenty degrees, then the water in the pond in the park down the street may have some ice on it—assuming of course that it does not have a water heater and/or is filled with salt water. We are in this case, using *statistics*—the science of building knowledge through the use of data, and *probability*—the science of measuring how likely an event is to occur, to build conclusions.

Even as youngsters, we are taught to believe with certainty that $1 + 1 = 2$.

We are, in these examples, drawing reasonable inferences based on observable data points and the accepted laws or rules of the environment. You could argue that the correlation between observations and predictions is something that forms our first lessons of life.

We live based on knowing the fundamental relationships between actions and activities (the variables) and the results (outcomes). If you speed and get caught by the police, for example, you will more than likely get a ticket. Similarly, if you eat a pound of bacon every morning for breakfast, you will more than likely gain weight, especially if you're lacking ways of expending the extra calories you consumed.

Both scenarios are examples of the equations of life and how current actions can lead to future and sometimes severe reactions or consequences. Despite the fact that one example dealt with the consequences of an action on your body (for example, sitting in jail to await a court date since when the police pulled you over for speeding, they discovered you also had ten unpaid parking tickets) while the other focuses on the consequences of an action on your life (eating too much bacon equals weight gain), they have tremendous similarities when viewed as a series of variables and outcomes.

The concept of equation is the foundation of PHC. The input variables in the evolving life equation of our future systems of PHC include your actions (A), your genome (G), and the environment (E) while the output is your unique health status (H). The view of your health becomes a simple statement of $H = f(A, G, E)$ in which "f" refers to the complex relationships of known and unknown that govern and define the interactions of these relatively simple concepts.

Easy to understand? For most of us, the answer is yes but with a few caveats. It is relatively easy, for example, to acknowledge the relationship of pedaling a bicycle and its forward movement. But how do the various movements we all make in our lives impact our future health status?

Scientists today, for example, believe that cancer is often the result of some environmental influence with a root cause and time and may have some linkage back to your genetic code. What's left to determine are variables that are most difficult to define, such as when that first renegade cell was created and what caused it to appear. And what was in the environment and the reactions within our genes and cells (or some other deeper level of data) that caused the transformation from "normal" to "abnormal?"

Add another ingredient in this murky mix—the untold power of connections. Each of the unique variables of our life equation form combinations that influence health outcomes. Counterbalancing the more than 25,000 genes scientists believe maintain some relevance in your life with the countless environments you could live in or around along with the almost infinite number of actions you could take and you get a glimpse of the research opportunities facing our future health care system.

To further muddy the waters, add the impact of geologic thinking— and the reality that events unfold over long periods of time—and the problem shifts from being arithmetic to geometric in depth. Yes, Einstein's laws of physics were wonderful and complex discoveries of how our world operates—at least according to several of the more critical relationships of time and space. However, these almost infinite collections of variables of living represent another and more complex set of issues I believe will tax every bit of creative intuition humans have to resolve.

Let's say, for example, you woke up this morning feeling perfectly fine and by dinner you felt ill. What happened during the day to cause this change? Clearly you and your body moved from one particular point on a timeline to another—shifting from the morning to late afternoon to evening. Along the way, you experienced a collection of events, which may have ranged from exposure to a virus floating around your environment to perhaps stubbing your toe. The collection of events that occurred throughout the day and at specific moments of time I have labeled as the *life variables*.

What are they and what values are critical to understand? The answers are not clear. What is important and what is simply "noise," or unrelated to any outcome—and what is noise today but eventually becomes critical later—is the single greatest challenge facing our scientific community searching for the clues and answers in the future systems of PHC.

But let's return again to our example of the life equation, with a shift this time to how the events occurring at one point in time can have a correlation to your health status at some later date. Could an action you took one day in the past have a causal relationship to an event that appears in your life twenty years later? And returning to an earlier question—could there be a relationship between receiving a speeding ticket today and your health status at some indeterminate time in the future? Unfortunately, and for reasons that are far outside of the scope of this book, the answer could be yes. But how can this be?

For a sense of the complexity of the answer assume the following: each of the variables of our life equation could have an impact that ranges from the nearly immediate to the long-term. Complicating matters is the fact that in each moment in time you introduced yet another set of variables with a corresponding set of additional forward relationships.

What is the result? During the course of our life you have defined a number of relationships that expand in a nearly geometric rate with each having the potential to cause cascading downstream events. And at their outset, some might even appear to have absolutely no relationship to the eventual outcome. So when they appear you are basically blinded and unaware that they could have represented a seminal moment in your life—and with tragic long-term consequences. Taking a loaded gun to your head and shooting will lead to an obvious and highly probable result—that is, you will die. But what about the stress you experienced in a failing marriage and its subtle impact on your immune system? Where will that "variable" lead?

This is, to me, an incredibly scary concept. Who would have thought that receiving a speeding ticket may have been a factor in the heart disease you experienced later in life? Was exposure to Agent Orange, for example, the cause of the cancer that appeared at some later date for a number of Vietnam vets?

While the premise sounds bizarre, the reality is not. All of the interdependent relationships housed within our life equation will no doubt conspire in some way to interfere with the mission and, eventually, the *mechanics* of your body.

The evolving answers to these life equation variables form the theory behind the newly emerging PHC system. When someone decided to populate our bodies with life and a vastly complicated network of cells, we shifted to a destiny of nearly infinite possibilities. Life is not as simple as we may like it to be, at least given today's level of knowledge.

So given this complexity where do we start in our quest to find the answers that will help ease us into a PHC system? The answer is simple: we will start by looking at ourselves. But don't expect to find too many easy answers.

Searching for Clues

Let's return to our earlier question: Why did Dana Reeve develop lung cancer? What linkage of data points in her life and within her own genome would have predicted the rise of cancer and its destructive impact on her health? Where was it in the timeline of her life equation that her cancer was introduced, only to carve its virulent growth trajectory?

Like any good detective novel, the ultimate answer is buried within the data points of her life. Clearly she shared a number of common characteristics with all of us. She was born, carried a collection of genes, and weaved her way through various environments, performing actions that helped to establish the state of her mechanical body at evolving points in time.

The first challenge in finding the answer to the why/when question is in defining Reeve's "Human Map"—the collection of internal data points (including the genome) that conspired to define her cancer. But how does a person find this data and then, once discovered, how do you establish the correlations in a world where each individual's reaction may vary based on the script of their genome? Solving the problem of 1 + 1 = 2 is easy to understand, the web of connections over time in the life equation are not. But it is a problem we have seen before in our movement to an era of scientific reasoning.

The questions of data and measurement are well documented in the research community—with the major issue facing almost all scientific discoveries being one of building a collection of unbiased data points that reinforce the "truth" of a theory. The most recent discoveries in the field of physics are being driven, for example, through the use of innovative experiments that allow us to observe new physical particles—and some of the smallest observable elements of matter. The data required to build the emerging applications of PHC will require no less of a focused effort and nearly limitless sources of information about the physical state of an individual over time and how they exist within the boundaries of environments.

Put aside the almost random collection of environments and environmental variables, and think for a moment of the messy starting point—our genes. Each of these genes has the potential to express either individually or in combination with others to form proteins that act as messengers that eventually define the health and disease status of an individual. How the impact of these genes unfolds over time—their *expression*—and the cases in which this expression is done incorrectly contains one of the world's largest data-gathering challenges.

So once you have this emerging collection of data points on our genes, the defined pathways of disease, and our various therapeutic approaches and individual reactions how do we know what is the best way of representing it? Understanding that our bodies are governed by the reactions of an equation is great on a theoretical level, but it raises a number of issues on the data capture side—along with a number of questions on the best way of bringing it back to the user.

The reality is that it is easy to get lost. Lacking a contextual framework—*and a point of reference*—it is easy to lose sight of the value of a particular piece of information. Receiving an LDL score on a blood test of 130 mg/dl in isolation has absolutely zero value to most of us. It is when you are given a piece of data and can evaluate its other relative information, for example contrasting a score of 130 mg/dl with changes over time or average "healthy" values, that it becomes important. With context and references you have the ability to shift data to knowledge and eventually integrate this knowledge into your actions.

But we have a major intellectual problem confronting our data analytics task beyond our simple measures of blood chemistry—the world of three and four dimensions. As living creatures we exist within a physical space (the three dimensions) and move through time (the fourth dimension). And the various systems of our bodies live within the physical laws of our world, having depth and connections that move from single data points to almost infinite complexity and interconnections. So how are we expected to place these various life equation variables within the context of our bodies? How do we establish the reference framework—and what will it look like?

Anyone know where we can find a good mapping program for the body?

Note

1. Final Mortality Statistics Report, National Center for Health Statistics, 1997–2003.

PART II

CHALLENGES OF DATA

Anyone can count the seeds in an apple, but only God can count the number of apples in a seed.

—ROBERT SCHULLER

THE MAPQUEST CORPORATION has made life for their countless users far easier. Their clever product is software that runs on the Internet and allows the user to indicate a starting point and final destination so MapQuest can build a set of electronic directions.

As many of us appreciate, a map is a requirement for an extended trip, with the country's road system representing a sometimes confusing set of alternatives when trying to get from one place to another. In less than a decade, MapQuest has demonstrated how the information-age version of the map can move far beyond the paper product, once the mainstay of travelers around the world. The MapQuest solution takes the map—a coordinate space that conforms to the landscape and roads of the land—and places it on your computer and within its immense powers to *transform and manage data.*

Why is MapQuest, or similar Internet mapping applications, better than the tried-and-true paper version we came to rely on over the years (and centuries) of mapmaking—and are also relevant to the systems of personalized health care (PHC)?

First on the list of reasons is the power to change. One of the things modern society has imposed on the landscape of the earth is the roads we use to go between one place and another. While our mountains, lakes, rivers, and coastlines remain constant (or at least generally so), the paths that we use to connect towns and houses are subject to growth and redevelopment. The beauty of our electronic maps is that they have the ability to dynamically change and be redefined based on this new and evolving information. While the paper version requires a new run of the printing press, the electronic substitute requires a simple refresh of an Internet browser.

MapQuest builds upon this concept of information flexibility in how it provides a set of directions through the most current information available on the roads between two locations. It even has the potential to include real-time data based on accidents and detours that may have occurred on the roads after they were built.

The next major advantage of this new form of mapping is in how the information is delivered to you. When you purchase a road atlas, you face an immediate limitation—its lack of portability. Sure, paper can be carried between locations. And clearly a map is not something designed to simply be housed in a set location. Maps often move around as their owner carries them from place to place as they travel from here to there.

The problem is that the information housed on the paper map requires that you have the ability to read and understand it—and become actively involved in finding the solutions to your tracking question. It requires your brain to come up with an answer, which in most cases involves picking a likely path between two locations or trying to figure out where you are. That is where the MapQuest-style solution wins yet another of its races with its paper predecessor.

As I'll discuss in Part III, the combination of electronic information and the processing power of a computer have resulted in countless interesting and innovative ideas. In the case of mapping, the combination of computer processing and information has made the task of figuring out how to move between locations a problem belonging to MapQuest, not you. If, for example, you prefer to avoid big highways, online Internet mapping applications can provide a mapping conclusion based on this new "parameter." The MapQuest map can also adapt to your needs thanks to a substantial number of supporting innovations from the world of engineering sciences, allowing you to view your maps on multiple devices and forms, including cell phones.

If you are still not convinced the paper-map industry is changing, take a look at some of the new cars rolling off production lines in Japan, Germany, or Detroit. In today's world, the concept of Internet mapping has gone even more high tech by introducing real-time navigation.

A global positioning system (GPS) responds by coordinating a car's location with a satellite somewhere in the sky. When the driver inputs data, such as the desired destination, into the GPS, the system can provide directions verbally, directing the driver to turn left in one hundred yards or instruct him to prepare to continue straight. The electronic map is moving in directions and at a speed that its paper competitors can't match.

Mapmaking, as you will come to appreciate, is also a critical element of the PHC system of the future and will define a development platform for a new generation of knowledge "utilities."

The Body and Infinity

The proposed *human map* is ultimately an evolution of an idea that builds upon the rich heritage of the early mapmakers, spanning Hippocrates in 400 BC to Craig Venter, Francis Collins, and his colleagues at the NIH and their work on the Human Genome Project in the late twentieth century. And given the evolving knowledge and general variation of our bodies, building the human map represents one of the more interesting problems our modern mapmakers have yet faced. Imagine how difficult it would be to move between two cities if, on any given day, you discovered the path from one city to the next was not the same as it was when you took the path yesterday.

This is the challenge ahead of us as we attempt to generalize the anatomy of our bodies and the intellectual issue for the health professions that work on us. The maps we once relied on to help navigate us through our cities and countryside, and even those created by interactive programs like MapQuest, enjoy the luxury of capturing the coordinates of a single place—the earth. And although we are constantly adding towns, roads, and houses, it remains confined to its single planetary surface.

Humans, however, are quite different. As you notice when you walk around any shopping mall, our world is filled with people of varying shapes and ages. And their resulting internal structures differ from one another, as well. Although we are all *Homo sapiens* and share a number of key similarities (like the types of internal organs, number of bones, etc.), we are not exactly the same on our insides. As any general surgeon can tell you, when a human body is opened, small surprises can be found in the final packaging. The realities of individual variation represent the first test for the human mapmaker. The next obstacle is in how much detail to include.

But what if each point on a map could drill down into a nearly infinite set of lower points? How would you define or visualize this coordinate space?

In a two-dimensional world, like that provided to you when you received the recommendations from MapQuest on how to travel from your home in, say, Chicago to a relative's home in Duluth, it is easy to follow the path between two points and the various right and left turns required on your journey. Moving to an "outer space" friendly version of MapQuest, you could imagine the same set of right and left turns given to you as you headed from Earth to Mars and then maybe to a moon of Jupiter. But imagine how hard the task becomes if for each set of recommendations, that is, the suggested left and right turns, you were forced to go deeper and deeper into your destination. In this case the directions for traveling from your home in Chicago to your relative in Duluth also had to include moving within your relative's house to a specific room on the second floor and a final destination on a chair in a bedroom. Now add to the complexity the possibility that the target chair may have been moving around while you created the map and was now located in a different room in the basement or had been reupholstered and now looked different. Each of these additions to the mapmaking challenge represents new levels of complexity in how to define destinations and would have become a nightmare for the software developers of MapQuest were they trying to build this new fictional version of the product. Welcome to the complexity challenge of the human map, where our emerging knowledge of even higher-level systems (e.g., a heart) can be subdivided into increasingly lower-level data representations. Our bodies are a complicated mixture of connections of systems, with almost infinite levels of depth.

And whether or not we like it, it is depth that defines our existence.

Start with the body. Dive into its collections of cells (our gross anatomy), individual cells, internal structures of a cell, the DNA, and a variety of lower and lower level components and you appreciate the wide expanse of the living organism. The challenge is in understanding how, where, and when to intervene if a problem occurs—and at what level the appropriate intervention should take place.

Is the best place to attack cancer at the level of the DNA, a cell, or the mass of the tumor? How far down you can go inside of our bodies with relative certainty is an interesting question, but one thing is clear: the mapping issues of the body are a long-term opportunity for a wide array of data miners.

The final challenge for our human mapmakers is the concept of aging and the body's evolution. We all generally understand that our bodies change in appearance as we move from childhood to our adult years, growing in size and filling in according to some programmed pattern. Why does this happen? And how is it controlled and at what level?

A powerful example of just how complicated even this simple question of growth in our bodies really is—and how even this basic activity seems to be broken into its own collection of independent maps—can be found in the surgery community and their approach to the challenges of managing craniofacial deformities.

Destiny

Performing a craniofacial surgery on a young child is a complex undertaking. The procedure requires a team of skilled professionals and countless hours of surgery. As most appreciate, surgery is typically the event of last recourse and should be given the potential it has for "collateral" damage—whether as a result of the analgesic impact on the brain and organ systems or the general invasion of the body. For a number of these craniofacial cases, taking the young child to the operating theater is a requirement if the child hopes to have a normal development—and the potential to realize the many talents contained within their young bodies. The question facing the surgeon thus becomes when to schedule the most appropriate time for these required operations.

Over the past few years, an interesting observation has been made on bone growth. It became clear that the developing bones of a young child would follow a growth path based on the underlying script contained within their genome. Were you to try and force fit a new shape, for example, the bones would at some later date realign themselves into the shape that their genes had decided they should be. It was as if their bones had an internal brain and decided that after the surgery was performed and the human intervention had resulted in a change in how they fit together they—the bones, that is—would retake control and reshape themselves in the way they decided was best. The bones were following their own mission-based driver.

Happily, the conclusion of this case study is positive. By recognizing the bones had a certain predestined quality to where they would align during their development phase, it became obvious that the more the surgeon interfered with the natural movements of the bones during this growth period, the more they simply exposed the child to the potential damages a surgery can bring.

So how should the surgeon handle this reality that their handiwork could be undone by some force other than their own hands—and completely outside of their control? The answer was that within the craniofacial surgery community, it became accepted that more is not always better, at least when it comes to children. The overwhelming opinion of the surgical community was to ensure the child was not harmed during these growth periods—and worry about the more cosmetic issues later.

This concept of internal missions is a complex and mysterious affair, which only underscores the intense integration housed within our bodies and how difficult it is to understand the depth and range of its potential.

The goal of the proposed human map is to provide the coordinate space to manage and house these expanding lower-level coordinates that will eventually be used to define the new systems of PHC. As our example in craniofacial surgery highlights, this new mapping question will no doubt establish a number of its own unique and novel approaches to how we represent data. How should you best characterize the growth patterns of bones within a child—and also account for the unique variations that occur among all of us?

Luckily, the mapping challenge is being helped by a number of discoveries in the diagnostic community with the advent of new and more powerful ways of exploring the inner reaches of the body. It is a set of technologies that have evolved quite a bit since their discoveries in the twentieth century. And that evolution has been fascinating.

The goal of Part II is to expose you to the reality of information—how society has changed its way of thinking about what constitutes important data points and how we are starting to establish ways of categorizing information. Recall the discussion on the life equation and the $H = f(A, G, E)$ model.

Get ready for data overload—but it is an overload that you will have to manage. Because while the life equation is an elegant and simple way of defining your health destiny, it masks what is an increasingly complex problem in the acquisition and organization of data: how to transform data to knowledge and action.

CHAPTER 3

UNCERTAINTY AND TRUTH

IN 1927, THE PHYSICIST Werner Heisenberg introduced the world to a radical theory on one of the newer physical laws of our universe. His idea came with a startling conclusion: the more we understood about our universe the more we became aware that it was an unpredictable and confusing place.

It had not been that way before, thanks to the work of scientists from Newton to Einstein and the evolving knowledge of classical physics. The apple fell from the tree, for example, and the laws of gravity would define a certain path (i.e., downward) and conclusion (i.e., hitting the ground).

Heisenberg accepted, as did all serious scientists of the day, that the laws of classical physics made it possible to predict the movement of a particle based on the knowledge of its location and its momentum. Heisenberg's assertion was that this predictability of outcome was not the case in the world of the quanta and the very small. In stark contrast to the physical universe described by Newton, the world of the quanta was governed by uncertainty, with no simple correlation of future state to action.

This question of certainty in outcomes is an analogous debate that haunts us today when dealing with the various cause-and-effect relationships in health care. Some people that smoke get cancer, others do not. Why does this happen?

And what is "truth," anyway? Let's start by acknowledging that the process of finding it is often a journey of continuous discovery. While technology has made it easier to communicate between distances and allows individuals to voice opinions in a way that was impossible in the pre-Internet era, it has not necessarily made it easier to figure out which point of view is correct.

We may have plenty of data, opinions, and interpretations on the facts of health and living but which of these are relevant and provide insight and should be included in an analysis of our health status? Having more, as the Internet has so aptly demonstrated, is not always better.

The first challenge we face in constructing our larger map of the body and in defining the relevant variables in our life equation is this issue—and understanding which pieces of information are right, wrong, relevant, and/or irrelevant—as we try to understand the relationship between perceived variables and outcomes. These are tough questions to answer and, as demonstrated by Vioxx (which we thought was a wonder drug when it first hit the market), may be subject to change over time (we later discovered Vioxx was a death sentence for certain people).

What would have happened, for example, were we to have discarded the theories of our early research community as they challenged the notion of how the heart worked or even the position of the earth within our solar system? Our history is filled with countless examples of ideas that are later disproved based on new data points and more thorough evaluations. We are, for better or worse, living largely in a world of uncertainty, and it is critical that we accept that our knowledge of life, our universe, and almost everything around us is limited— and sometimes wrong. While incredibly clever animals, we are nowhere near as smart as we would like to believe—and especially so when it comes to the issues of how our bodies really work.

Changing your mind is therefore not only a good thing to do, it also demonstrates that you are still thinking.

Building Confidence

At the time when Ken Olsen, who had built a career through a combination of engineering excellence and vision, made that now infamous prediction in a 1977 meeting of the World Future Society in Boston that "there is no reason anyone would want a computer in their home," few people had room to argue with him.

As the founder and CEO of the one of the most powerful and innovative computer companies of the day, he was in a position to know. And along with his position of leadership in the industry, he had an absolutely outstanding pedigree.

An MIT graduate, Olsen enjoyed a career that included a stint at the illustrious Lincoln Labs, one of the world's great engineering centers. He was, by all accounts, as closely connected to the future of computing as anyone in the industry—with the company he founded, the Digital Equipment Corporation (DEC), accepted as one of the market's innovative leaders.

Ken Olsen was quite simply an "expert."

Yet his prediction on the future of the computer in the home was completely wrong. Computers are today a widely accepted and ubiquitous utility in everything from business to entertainment, a reality that became apparent within ten years of Olsen's 1977 prediction. And they have continued their evolution into ever smaller forms and functions and can be found everywhere from your desktop to inside your refrigerator and car.

The underlying message of this example is that people should be careful before they decide on what is true and accurate. How, for example, do we know that our use of cell phones is safe and that we can expect no long-term damage to our ears, brains, or other body parts?

The answer is that we don't.

One of the conundrums in defining truth is that we have created an almost adversarial system of interests in which it is becoming increasingly difficult to determine if the presentation of information is coming through without bias or interpretation—or worse yet, is being intentionally misrepresented. Another point to remember is this: what society currently accepts as a guiding law may one day be proven to have been just another bad idea based on a poor interpretation of data.

Figure 3.1 indicates just how difficult this even simple task could become.

Consider the ideal scenario on the left, in what I have labeled as the "Optimal Knowledge Discovery Curve," or the generally hoped-for discovery path. In this graph we move through time gaining increasing confidence in a statement (or rather, a data point) from a start of zero reliability to almost 100 percent.

The graph on the right side of figure 3.1 illustrates a path to avoid.

The premise is a simple one—you start believing on Day x that some statement is correct, or at least has a reasonably high confidence score. But on Day x + y new information appears shifting your confidence in the statement lower, or the proverbial one step forward, three steps backward. How do you incorporate that type of statement of fact within your own thinking—or how do you use it as the basis for reaching some conclusion? The answer is that it is almost impossible, at least if you try to use any rational approach to building your answer.

Along with my earlier question on cell phones, are we also sure that the use of vitamin C as a nutritional supplement is good for our health? And if it is, is it good for everyone and in the same way? As strange as it may seem, our experience with Vioxx would suggest that the answer is no.

Figure 3.1. Discovery and Confidence Factors

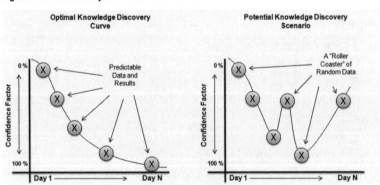

Knowing the Source

Constructed through a series of data points that correspond to the coordinates of the earth, the recommendations of MapQuest have a certain unquestioned elegance. The earth is something we can all touch and feel. And the "truth" of the earth is relatively easy to grasp, at least in terms of its dimensions. We live on it and its surface is the playing field of our lives.

But how do we define the truth of the body? On one level, these questions have a simple set of answers. If you are alive, and I will assume you are since you are reading this book, then you can clearly discover some of the more basic signs of your existence, such as your pulse and the fact you are breathing and so on. These high-level data points establish a level of confidence that is difficult to dispute.

Humans are the result of millions of years of evolutionary forces but we have conformed to certain assumptions of biological life. The need to feed our bodies, whether through breathing or eating, is an example of one of the most basic.

Scientists, however, have defined an increasing number of new data points, many of which appear confusing or hidden within a broader collection of information resources. Separating fact from fiction is hard enough but doing so when also parsing through the body's often confusing data points in an attempt to define the patterns of life that will impact your health is practically mind-boggling. Is an HDL level of 60 mg/dl good to have, for example? And what is a fractionated lipid?

When I introduced the life equation I established a relatively simple function that showed the relationship of variables to an outcome. Health status, as suggested then, was a function (or equation) of the individual's environment, their internal life script (or genome), and their actions.

Simple enough if you think about it as related to one moment in time, but infinitely complex when you discussed its potential impacts moving from one time to another. It's now time to introduce the next level of complexity that you will need to understand and the foundation for the life equation—the selection of the relevant variables.

Where do we start this journey? Let's begin with a single point. When a point appears in isolation it is at least easy to quantify—and we may be able to connect it to either some downstream or immediate event. Alcohol is an example of a single data point that as a poison can cause immediate problems within the body in addition to its potential to inflict long-term damage.

Now shift that single point, as highlighted in figure 3.2, and place it within a broader collection of other points, many of which we believe represent simple background noise. By noise, we are implying that they have absolutely no relevance to an end state—at least given today's knowledge. The challenge is now how to identify what is clearly relevant and connected—which are highlighted by the linear connection of the circled "1s" in figure 3.2—from those data points that have absolutely no bearing on health outcome. One of the striking examples of these causal relationships, for example, is between the drug acetaminophen (Tylenol) and alcohol.

The reality is that within the context of any moment in time, your body is exposed to an almost countless array of variables or impacts. Some you can control (like how much sleep you get, whether you exercise, whether your job is stressful), while others simply appear in the environment (like the quality of water you drink or the air you breath). However, they all share something in common: they all either conspire to or succeed in producing some novel effect that could range from practically nothing to death.

In isolation, and taken according to directions, Tylenol will, for example, do almost exactly what it was designed to do. Putting aside the Vioxx Impact—that any individual's reaction to Tylenol may not be the same as another's—we now also understand that when ingested with alcohol, Tylenol may have a long-term negative impact on our liver. And even this starts with the reality Tylenol by itself can be deadly.

A 2005 study[1] by Ann Larson of the University of Washington highlighted just how dramatic of an impact Tylenol (and more generally, acetaminophen) had on liver failure. In 1998, the first year of the study, the number of liver failures caused by acetaminophen was

Figure 3.2. Defining Relevancy

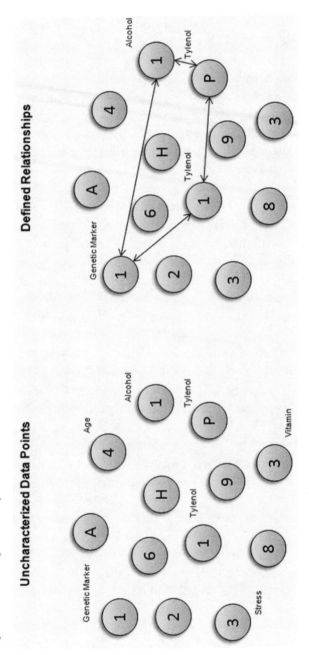

28 percent. By the end of the study period in 2003 that number had risen to 51 percent.

It turns out that our bodies can be relatively sensitive to the accumulation of acetaminophen, with long-term use (of say 7.5g, with the recommended dose being 4g) potentially leading to liver toxicity. This reality of the changing nature of outcomes based on exposure over time highlights another of the major challenges of our emerging knowledge of the mission variables of health and how a relatively benign act (taking Tylenol) can evolve and lead to devastating conclusions.

So the next time you have been drinking—and may have had more than you should have, which caused a nasty and throbbing headache—probably the last thing you should add to the mix of chemicals in your body is too much Tylenol. Unless, that is, you are anxious to be added to the list of acetaminophen-induced liver failures. The Larson study should have been a wakeup call for everyone that believes that "if you can buy it on the shelf of a grocery store" it must be safe.

So what about all of those sugar-laden breakfast cereals? Do they have any relationship to the rising tide of Type II diabetes?

One thing is perfectly clear. Almost none of us really understand how the mix of chemical touch points in our environment can kill us, with the most complicated part of the equation being that it may not happen today, next month, or even next year. It is frightening to consider the potential interactions of other activities in our lives and how little we know today of their downstream relationships. Were we living in an age of an integrated system of PHC, theoretically people would have at least had the knowledge that large quantities of Tylenol and your liver don't mix—which would have been a great start.

Now it's time to make the problem a bit more difficult by putting this data problem in the context of reality. Life is filled with countless exposures, so rarely do we find ourselves with a simple one-to-one relationship of actions and environment to outcomes. Our bodies are also filled with their own collections of seemingly endless data points that are part of the ultimate evaluation process.

When we described the general life equation, we established a model for conceptualizing the practices of PHC. Health outcomes became a function of the actions of an individual, their genome, and the surrounding environment. The complexity of this equation is compounded by the shifting timeline of our lives and the potential of an individual data point—the specific variable—to impose different end results over different times. Unfortunately for us this sea of data points becomes again more complex as we:

- **Expand our knowledge of what is important and relevant.** Are there new information points that we should be adding to the mix of our life equation that have potential immediate or long-term connections? Was exposure to a certain strain of the flu, for example, a predictor of some later health condition?
- **Increase our knowledge of genetic relationships.** The connection of a health outcome will no doubt involve a correlation of a variety of genes and genetic expressions. We know, for example, that the BRCA1 and BRCA2 genes are relevant to the prediction of breast cancer. What causes these and other damaging genes to express?
- **Increase our knowledge of the Gene–Cell–System architecture.** The body represents a combination of puzzle pieces and puzzles, with the DNA in our cells clearly playing a vital role. As we discover more about the relationship of our body's genetic infrastructure to our body will that change our view of how to attack certain health conditions—and establish the best point of intervention?
- **Recognize the data-collection problem as being time-sensitive.** We are living in a dynamic, rich environment that is governed by the movement of time. At what time points do we slice our data analysis to determine patterns and relationships?

The ultimate impact of these questions is that we have an immense data-gathering task ahead of us and a need to obtain greater clarity in our search for answers. What will be the source of this data? The answer is our bodies and environment and through data-harvesting approaches that span things as simple as taking your pulse, to the complex discoveries of the X-ray, the MRI, and the evolving discoveries in physics. The twentieth century was a rich period of discovery for our data-mining colleagues, with the invention of a host of new technologies becoming the new stage of discovery for medicine.

Note

1. Anne M. Larson et al., "Acetaminophen-induced acute liver failure: Results of a United States multicenter, prospective study," *Hepatology* 42, no. 6 (December 2005): 1364–72.

CHAPTER 4

THE DATA HARVEST

NOT MANY PEOPLE remember the Adrian X-Ray Company. From their headquarters in Milwaukee, Wisconsin, they were one of the early pioneers in the data-mining field. Set your calendars back to the early twentieth century for a few clues to their identity.

Adrian's product was a simple combination of emerging technologies, including an X-ray and a fluoroscope.

The shoe industry has always been competitive. It was no accident, therefore, that in the 1930s, shoe stores would be one of the first industrial groups outside of medicine to embrace the potential values of the X-ray. For the first time in history customers who used the shoe-fitting fluoroscope had an opportunity to watch their toes wiggle and see how well their shoe fit the contours of their foot inside of their shoe as they wore them. It was a science fiction–like event that started with good intentions.

Adrian had hit a home run with its customers, or at least it appeared that way.

Given these advantages, the obvious question is, why was the shoe-fitting X-ray forcefully taken off the market starting in the 1950s? To understand the answer we will need to dive into our body's mechanics.

The cells of our bodies are extremely sensitive little machines. Anyone who has at least a passing knowledge of biology likely stands in awe of the complex interactions taking place within each of their walls. From the control center of the nucleus, which houses our

DNA, to the membrane, the cell comes with its own collection of internal functions and interactions that add to the already complicated mixture of systems we have in our bodies.

And here is the problem for Adrian. X-rays, it turns out, have the potential to damage a cell's internal structure and produce a number of unfortunate downstream events, with one of the worst being cancer. But X-rays also have a tendency that is not surprising of any mission-driven variable—they can have an impact, but it is not always clear when their results will be felt or how.

The reality is that X-rays represent the ultimate double-edged sword. On one hand they provide tremendous value in showing us something that, lacking technology, we would be unable to see. The appeal of seeing a closely fitting shoe, or knowing that a bone was actually broken, is strong. Yet on the other hand we were becoming aware, by the time the Adrian product appeared on the markets in the 1950s, that there was a connection between X-ray exposure and cancer. Was the correlation clear?

The answer would require a bit of digging and was forcing us to begin thinking about our bodies and the relation of our environment and actions to a physical condition in ways that we had not done in previous generations. Remember that in Osler's day and before, the idea of disease was often mysterious, with little understanding of how these various disease states appeared. And this understanding was clearly not at the level of cell interaction (or damage) as subtly caused by the X-ray.

Now enter the age of biochemistry. In our emerging world of the twentieth century we were beginning to appreciate the relationship of these tiny cells in our bodies to the complex environment of our various body systems—and the potential for there to be a relationship of these systems and outcomes to their surroundings. We later added even further and deeper knowledge of genetics and how these systems were governed by an underlying script that was somehow included in absolutely every corner of our bodies.

Adrian and their shoe-fitting fluoroscope had fortunately (for us as consumers that is) entered a period of our history where we were starting to apply a stronger scientific rationale to the understanding of problems. Where in the earlier days of the Mayans a lack of rain may have been viewed as some form of displeasure by the gods, we were by the middle of the twentieth century beginning to use reasoning based on what we understood of the physical laws of our bodies to solve our problems. Unfortunately for Adrian, the first indication that there may be a potential problem with X-rays was noticed almost immediately after their discovery in the late days of the nineteenth century.

While it may have taken a few decades longer than it should have, by the 1950s we understood that overexposure to X-rays had a strong correlation to cancer. And the Adrian device was using a fair amount of X-ray power to create a moving picture of its customer's toes.

No one—then or now—should assume that the leadership of Adrian had intended on causing an increase in cancer in the users of its product. Adrian was simply another example of a firm that was acting ahead of our society's accepted knowledge, with no comprehension of the long-term impact of its product on its customers. Thalidomide, Vioxx, and the shoe-fitting X-ray are all examples of how easily we can make mistakes with products—and how hard it can be to understand the consequences of our actions.

Clearly the mechanical foundation of our bodies is important, but we also need to base our actions using a deeper appreciation for the complexity and power of our personal life equation and our body's mission. Who would have thought that having your toes checked at the shoe store in the 1940s could have resulted in cancer at some later date? You can bet that none of the people who used the Adrian shoe-fitting fluoroscope did.

They were, after all, only visiting a shoe store.

So how do we ever know if an environment is safe for us?

To begin answering this question, we will need more advanced ways of defining the data points that populate our human map. The birth of the X-ray was a hint of the future, although this time it was not being used in the shoe industry, or at least it did not start that way. The pace of innovation along the way has been staggering.

Looking Inside the Body

In 1895, Wilhelm Roentgen introduced the world to the potential of the X-ray through an innovative experiment that allowed us to visualize past flesh into the bones of his hand. With the Roentgen X-ray we could for the first time in our history see the inside of the living human.

Given our current understanding of anatomy, it is hard to believe that prior to the discovery of the X-ray our bodies were often shrouded in mystery. We obviously understood something about their internal structures—the history of this field is filled with interesting interpretations of our body's various systems based on knowledge gained through dissection. Yet I would argue that more than being a creative addition in our quest for the perfect roadmap of the body, the ultimate miracle of X-ray was how it opened a door to a new way of thinking.

If you can see inside the living body, what would you now look for? Would you try to identify patterns of disease and attack them before they reached their most virulent stage?

The X-ray was one of those sea-changing events of history that, during the ensuing years of the twentieth century, evolved from simple collections of black-and-white images to rich three-dimensional pictures that depicted movement and function. We could now witness the machine of our bodies in action—and do it while our bodies were still alive.

The next data question is more basic—what is the fuel of life that turns our collection of elements and systems into a living and breathing organism? We can see the inside but what makes it work? The answer is simple: chemistry and our genome.

Powering the Machine

Our bodies operate through an array of chemical interactions—spanning the mining of energy from glucose to the firing of neurons to controlling thought. But chemistry is a science with a long history that has been constrained by at least one stark reality—it is hard to explore the structures of the elements lacking the technology to visualize their inner depths.

The X-ray, while valuable in providing a snapshot of the larger structures of the body, would not help much in our grasp of the chemical world. Chemistry lives within the world of the very small, with the interactions of substances taking place in a space generally beyond our sight. It may be obvious, for example, that when you mix two chemicals together that you will achieve some type of reaction. But how does that reaction occur?

Between the Greek philosopher Democritus (460–370 BC) and the modern world, society witnessed a number of interesting experiments, with the critical breakthrough in our thinking—and the birth of the scientific platforms that later helped define our modern era—appearing during the eighteenth century. It was during this period that advances in our understanding of cells, and the old ideas on infectious diseases, were replaced with knowledge in microbiology and bacteriology.

The quantum leap in value came with the growth of our knowledge in pharmacology and our appreciation that specific drugs could be used to treat disease—with the most obvious being the growth of antibiotics and their abilities to confront the ravages of a number of bacteria-based disorders.

The next level of discovery changed the meaning of data forever and it came from the fields of biochemistry and biophysics. It is known as the genome.

The Age of the Genome

The genome is one of those elegant products of creation that is both striking in its simplicity yet incredibly complex in its function. Housing over 3 billion chemical pairs and constructed through a seemingly endless chain of connections, the human genome is one of the profound mysteries of our time.

Where does the genome fit in our lives? As anyone who has watched an episode of *CSI: Crime Scene Investigation* knows, genetic fingerprints have become an increasingly popular way of linking suspects to a crime and crime scene. We also understand that certain health conditions have a relationship back to our genes. Huntington's disease is one of the best known; the emerging knowledge of genetic markers for cancer is one of the newest and for many the most frightening.

The process of moving from the conceptual model of the genome—our combination of forty-six chromosomes and the more than 25,000 genes—to its physical map was an interesting trail that moved from the early work of Mendel to the innovative use of technology and theoretical constructs by James Watson, Francis Crick, and Rosalind Franklin.

We need to turn the clock back to the 1950s to understand the roots of science's recent success, where one of the most exciting intellectual races of the era was the race to decode the genetic architecture. The winners (Crick and Watson of Cambridge University and Franklin of Kings College) used the results of an experiment with X-ray diffraction combined with their own theoretical insights to uncover the missing piece of the puzzle. The end product of their victory, the knowledge of the double helix structure of our DNA, set the stage for a new era of gene-based discovery.

Why did it take almost another forty years before we began the gene-mapping project and the effort to codify the human genome? The answer can be found in technology—or rather a lack of the right kind. But that was about to change.

One of the more popular books of the recent era discusses a technical innovation, genetic cloning, that could be used to amplify the genetic structure of a dinosaur. The question raised by Michael Crichton in his novel, *Jurassic Park* (1990), was whether a snippet of a DNA sample could be used to rebuild a long since extinct dinosaur. The success of the book (and later movie) raised the public awareness of the potential of the genome along with a few interesting questions. Could we, for example, decode the individual life script of a single individual's genetic structure?

The answer to this question would require its own revolutions in technology—including the evolution of the polymerase chain reaction (PCR) and the power to amplify DNA. While Watson provided us with the general truth that our genome had a set of vocabularies to be read, the later efforts of the Human Genome Project sponsored by the National Institutes of Health (and pushed along by the Celera Corporation) helped provide the basic dictionary and knowledge that a legion of new scientific research would be required to uncover the more general screenplay.

And it has opened up an exciting future—the possibility of predicting a later stage of health based on the knowledge of our genetic script and, more simply, the ability to match the DNA of an individual with known genetic markers to aid in the diagnostic and therapeutic process. The most common example of this new line of thinking is the rise of pharmacogenomics—the science of defining how a specific individual will react to a specific medication.

Where in the past we typically thought of and delivered therapies through a "one-size-fits-all" model, the emerging pharmacogenomics therapies will be targeted to your specific genetic makeup and/or the specific genetic makeup of the disease. It is an exciting future enabled by the cumulative revolutions of the genome and the assumption that we have the ability to define a broader collection of data points on each of us and the disease conditions that affect our bodies.

But first a reality check—building this future will not be easy. As you may have guessed, moving from many models to one model will require a level of data and a way of understanding that we don't necessarily have in great supply today. How will we start?

Simple. We will start by creating some really interesting maps. So what would a map of you (or me) look like?

CHAPTER 5

BUILDING HUMAN MAPS

A LMOST ALL PEOPLE are born with two kidneys. When healthy, our kidneys filter through roughly two hundred quarts of blood producing nearly two quarts of waste products each day. In similar fashion, we have a heart, brain, and variety of other organ systems connected through a vast circulatory and nervous system—the electrical and chemical pathways of our bodies—in what is a striking balance of biological elegance.

It is the interaction of these and other systems that eventually defines our physical selves and forms the basis for whether we are healthy or are suffering from disease. Although this may not seem the case, scientists are really just beginning to scratch the surface on what we understand of our body's vast and interconnected systems. The mapping of our bodies—ranging from the fundamental questions of how we define the system components (e.g., an organ through a cell), how we measure appropriate values (e.g., glucose balance) and last, how we catalog this information—provide a major thread in the convergence leading to a system of personalized health care (PHC).

The difficulty in finding and describing these data points, in defining and building the human map, involve questions ranging from the location of the various parts to characterizing the interactions of our bodies at a cellular level and below. It is a complicated set of questions built upon a number of fundamental truths: We are living organisms who have a number of requirements to sustain life. We need to eat to build energy, we have a waste removal and repair process, and we age.

How complicated is the mapping challenge? You car has some clues on that future.

Living in 3-D

When you sit in the driver's seat of your car, turn the ignition, and drive away, you are probably unaware of the volumes of complex information the car is managing for you—a vast expanse of cabling controls this clever integration of brute force explosions and electronic sensors. But the final packaging of today's vehicles represents more than simply an example of great manufacturing ideas. They also highlight another element of data representation that has become critical to industry: visualization and modeling. Where's the connection?

Our modern cars are subject to a tremendous number of design constraints. Predicting its curbside appeal and ensuring it will drive effectively while meeting the various regulations on performance and safety defined by the government are difficult undertakings that are primarily achieved through the use of modeling systems—or computer-aided design (CAD).

Computers and CAD programs are being used by countless engineers and designers to model how a car will look, perform on the road, and, eventually, be manufactured. CAD has defined the process for creating a new generation of products and represents a set of tools that almost everyone in the industrial world understands. So, long before you sat in your car and drove away, someone had "driven" the equivalent of your car in a CAD environment and simulated your driving experience.

How will this same level of thinking enter health care and impact the growth of our human map?

Think for a moment of the environment facing the engineers working on the CAD systems and your car. Their models were built using three-dimensional structures—not simply the complex 2-D images provided by an X-ray. The car's engine, its physical structure, and the way the passenger and driver would fit within the car's contours were all problems that they could visualize within the 3-D space of the CAD's virtual world.

How do you create a more accurate picture of the rich world of the body's systems? The answer to this question was about to come from an unlikely company—at least for most of us that knew some of their more popular activities. They were founded in 1897 as the Gramophone Company and were primarily in the record business. We now know them as EMI.

EMI did something in 1972 that was about to build one of the more important pillars in our movement to PHC. They introduced the world to computed tomography (CT) and set the stage for a 3-D revolution in medicine.

CT was born without the usual fanfare normally given a major discovery. There were no parades and definitely not the round of talk-show appearances that have come to define breakthroughs in this country for its inventors. The CT went largely unnoticed for a number of reasons, with one of the biggest being the rather crude state of its product. It took several days to acquire the raw data for a single image and several more after that to reconstruct that single image into something the person could see. It also lacked the clarity that was found in the standard X-ray.

Why would anyone, for example, choose to undergo a CT when the X-ray offered far better resolution? The answer was that although the original CT clearly had a number of limitations, it proved to be a proverbial window to a new world, the 3-D space of our bodies.

Godfrey Hounsfield and Alan Cormack had started a revolution in body modeling.

Since Hounsfield's invention, the pace of innovation that has occurred in the diagnostics industry is staggering. Borrowing a technology discovery from the military community, we can now use sound waves to capture the moving image of a fetus. We have also learned how to excite our cells to an atomic level to create the miraculous images of the MRI, and, through the use of chemical markers, to view the systems of our body in action.

The resulting impact of these innovations is that we have moved from the flattened view of our bodies pioneered by Roentgen to the world of three dimensions, with the ability to see the inside of the body and its various systems without performing a physical dissection. We can now watch the living organism in the depth of its 3-D space.

Visualizing Motion

When the X-ray was discovered by Roentgen, it revolutionized the way people thought about the body and provided a view of its mechanics that had long been shrouded in mystery. Magnetic resonance imaging (MRI) provides another venue for peering inside of us and is based on a completely different way of taking a snapshot—a focus on the physics of an individual cell.

The theory behind the MRI comes straight out of a basic textbook and involves the use of extremely powerful magnets, a radio frequency pulse, and the rules of nuclear physics (that is, the properties of protons) to create an image of the body. So, how does this address the question of motion—or provide us with the ability to watch the body in action?

One of the more creative early efforts to visualize motion of the body's internal architecture was an invention by Drs. Elias Zerhouni, Elliot McVeigh, and several colleagues on a technique known as MRI tagging. Without diving into the technical details of the process, let me summarize it by saying simply that MRI tagging provided a noninvasive way of capturing and displaying motion in the patient's heart, which had previously represented one of the "big" problems of medicine.

Let's assume, for example, that you suffer from an early stage of cardiac disease. Through the technologies of MRI tagging, doctors could obtain a visual representation of your heart's muscles that could show early signs of damage without surgically entering your body. You could, in essence, sit back and watch your heart beat on a monitor and even track the progress of your heart's muscles in near real time, highlighting problems with your muscles that were previously hidden by an inability to see inside of the living human in action.

We had definitely moved a few conceptual miles ahead of the Roentgen discovery and the flat and static world of white-on-black images of X-ray. The heart is a dynamic, three-dimensional machine, and MRI tagging provided a way of watching it move as part of the body's larger system infrastructure.

MRI tagging was ultimately a revolution in thinking. The concepts introduced by Zerhouni, McVeigh, and their colleagues were early examples of how to visualize the dynamic elements of our body through the use of noninvasive technologies—and simply the start of yet another information race in medicine.

The pace of innovation since their discovery has been intense. Thanks to our friends in the field of nuclear medicine, we can watch blood flow and the cells fire in the brain in ways that were beyond the imagination of the physician working on your relatives in the nineteenth century.

Where do we go next? Luckily for us, the next major steps in the human map pursuit were taken by the National Institutes of Health (NIH) and its substantial community of scientists and academic partners. They came to the problem with an outstanding pedigree and commitment. They were, in the end, successful in their leadership of two incredibly complex tasks.

The Modern Body Conquests

Two of the most data-rich projects of the twentieth century were the catalogs of the human body developed by the National Institutes of Health through the Visible Human (VHP) and the Human Genome Projects (HGP). Representing the combined talents of an army of scientists, these efforts were a milestone for the emerging human map and took the success of the X-ray and the development of the 3-D model to the broader world of medical research—and these projects took entirely different paths in the same direction.

VHP was designed to provide the world's research community with a computer model of human anatomy created through a slice-by-slice image reconstruction of image "pictures." It was a painstaking and intricate task calling for a careful process of dissection and a number of images and photographs made from a male and female cadaver. The VHP, similar to the CAD programs of our car manufacturers, was looking at the bodies' three-dimensional world.

HGP had an equally ambitious goal: create a comprehensive picture of the human gene map through a reading of each of the unique genes contained within a selected donor genome. HGP, following the innovations of Watson and the discovery of the DNA's double helix, was looking at the lower-level mechanics of our cells.

VHP and HGP were also, by default, addressing the fundamental questions of how to map the human body and, more critically, establish the research base for our movement to the one-to-one systems of PHC.

The NIH was not alone in its pursuit of a broad mapping solution— the search for maps has in fact been one of the technical and intellectual quests of the ages. The early explorers, with the legendary Lewis and Clark expedition as one of the more powerful examples, demonstrated the power mapmaking has for pushing society ahead. But these newer human maps contained, as the NIH understood better than most, a number of issues that early mapmakers did not have to face, with the most obvious being that of dimension and the messy qualities of living organisms.

As we discussed with MapQuest, most mapmaking projects are focused on representations of the topological landscape of a particular place through an accurate and relevant set of measurements. When measuring the distance between one town and another, we tend to use feet/meters to gauge distances. An interesting although totally useless measure would be to suggest that one town is twelve ounces from another. The point is that for each map we define a measurement that is appropriate for describing its physical dimension.

So what are these critical measurements for the body, and are they flexible and sophisticated enough to accurately measure different bodies? As you can imagine, this is a question that will be answered differently based on the depth of the focal point—that is, how far down into the various systems of the body you have entered—and the type of system you are representing. A brain, for example, houses a vital control function that links how other systems work to, in some cases, specific physical points of the brain's 3-D space. The heart, in contrast, works more like a traditional pump as its muscles create force and push and pull the blood in our bodies through the vascular network.

Among the many other mapping issues of the body is the requirement to recognize that it moves through time and has a natural and somewhat predictable life and death cycle. It also mimics a machine in that it performs functions in concert—moving your finger involves a combination of muscle movements, dexterity of the joint, control of your brain, the movement of signals through your nerves, the feeding of the whole system through your vascular structure, and finally a way of healing and repairing itself.

But along with being a machine, our bodies are also like one big chemistry experiment—alter a value here and there and you may have a mess on your hands. Remember Love Canal and the unfortunate chemical mess created by the Hooker Chemical Company? You can bet that the residents of this small neighborhood outside of Niagara Falls had no idea that they were living in a chemical lab. And finally, and mysteriously through the miracles of evolution, the machines of our bodies operate with a precise set of balances that scientists are only now beginning to appreciate—and increasingly have the technology to measure.

So where do you start building this human map? A great place to frame this discussion is by looking at a map of the brain. Assume, as a starting point, that you are about to operate on a patient with a deeply rooted tumor.

The brain is the body's control center, housing the endpoints for a vast number of downstream linkages that monitor everything from sensory activities to our consciousness. Surgery on it is a complicated, risky undertaking with a number of potentially dangerous immediate and long-term consequences for the patient.

One of the starting points to this search of the brain's complexity involves the creation of a functional map—a solution that highlights another of the vast research questions our body-mapping projects face. Removing an unwanted growth from your finger, for example, has nowhere near the complications or downstream impacts that a similar procedure on your brain would entail.

To solve that shortcoming—and to attack the example of that deeply rooted tumor—there exists a need to define a different type of overlay, one that relates functional control (e.g., the sense of smell, the control of your right hand, the ability to think abstractly, etc.) to specific areas within the brain's 3-D space. But it introduces a different set of questions for the mapping community to answer.

Although our bodies are generally constructed using the same sets of parts (206 bones, two kidneys, one heart, etc.), humans are not necessarily built with each of these parts in exactly the same location or size. In general, this difference has no impact on people when it comes to the average surgery, but the story changes when the topic is the brain.

Mapping the Brain

If each brain possesses slight differences from one another, how can we construct a relevant set of coordinates that will travel from one brain to another? The answer is through the process of "normalization," which represents a mixture of computer science and mathematics and the creation of a system of standard measurements. The concept of standard "coordinates" is something we all use, often unknowingly, when we travel from one place to another. People tend to expect the distances between points A and B on a map will be the same each time they embark on the same trip, following the same path.

The notion of a normalized space based on coordinates provides the same level of assurance to our brain surgery colleagues. The normalization process gives the surgeon the ability to effectively line up their patient's brain with a collection of standard coordinates—morphing one to another and aligning their function. Through this alignment of function and space, the surgeon can determine how tinkering with one area of the brain (i.e., cutting here or there) may interfere with the patient's quality of life. Would you knowingly cut through an area around a tumor if you knew that by doing so you would cause blindness? The answer is no, or at least you should be, if you—the patient's surgeon—are worried about the quality of life of the patient after the operation is completed.

The combination of the *visualization* of the tumor's location—that is, the computer-generated 3-D view of the mass of the tumor and the brain—combined with the now normalized functional map, provides the surgeon with a set of resources far beyond what would have been found on a piece of paper. And through the integration of a number of other technical solutions empowered by the general revolution of the computer industry, the surgeon can bring that new knowledge directly into the operating theater and use it while performing the surgery on the patient.

So why is this finding—the ability to visualize a tumor and understand the surrounding function of the brain—important to the practices of PHC? The answer is that it helps us understand and work with individual variations in how we treat disease. Cutting a tumor out of a brain, it turns out, is not exactly the same from one person to another.

Imagine if the map between New York City and Boston were different for every person who planned a trip between these two cities. This is exactly the problem facing our brain surgery colleagues—and why the rise of the brain map is a critical marker for our future systems of health care. No, we are not all the same inside. And yes, you definitely want the surgeon cutting into your brain knowing that your brain has some variation from the last case she had.

But where will we go next? The answer is obvious, especially if you were one of the emerging gene data miners that were driving HGP—you turn your focus inward and begin exploring the mechanics of the cell at the level where the functional map was originally defined. The brain, like all of the organ systems, was a product of its DNA and the genome.

But as the members of the HGP understood early on, this initial set of goals—to identify the approximately 25,000 genes in the human DNA—was simply the start of the race. We may know, as a result of the HGP effort, the basic alphabet of our DNA, but next we need to understand the language, sentences, paragraphs, and books that this DNA describes.

And how do we put this new vocabulary within the context of a living universe, in which time sets the stage for change? Yes, we understand that the human genome contains over 3 billion base pairs. But we are also aware that a gene is only part of the story and maintains a complex set of relationships with other genes and proteins as a start. The questions are immense, to say the least.

Where do we go next?

CHAPTER 6

THE NEW MINERS

ONE THING IS CLEAR: the Visible Human Project (VHP) and the Human Genome Project (HGP) were an inflection point for the data-management community and a major success for the National Institutes of Health (NIH), the U.S. government, and the world's research enterprises.

But forget the fundamental value these projects provided in collecting massive amounts of raw image and genetic data and placing that data on computer-readable devices, which effectively translated into building an open market for research and development.

Also forget that they were only the small first step in what would later be a much larger data-acquisition program that invited the medical community to start considering areas of research and development at lower levels and increasing depths of complexity.

Last, forget that human genes serve as the library and construction surveyors for our bodies, thereby representing one of the most critical discoveries of our scientific era.

More than these tangible values, VHP and HGP are invaluable for an entirely different reason. They represent a general barometer of changing pressures in the data world of health. For an idea of how much of a change this was, simply think of where the research community had moved in just a few years.

Almost all of the early focus in the health-information industry was on record keeping and had one repeating mantra: schedule, treat, and bill. So while we had a digital revolution in health care, it was being led primarily by administrators, which is not necessarily bad but is clearly not the whole data story. Economic data may be good for understanding and projecting cost curves but it does not provide much of a platform for basic science research—or at least for those interested in the fundamental connections of our actions to how we can influence disease and health.

The net was that most people rarely thought about medicine as an area of rich data problems. Yes, some people "got it" and it was an exciting area of R&D for the small community of scientists in the medical informatics community—whose work was largely outside of the mainstream of large diagnostic systems (i.e., complex hardware) and chemistry.

The data-mining landscape changed dramatically when the community of researchers driving the VHP and HGP showed up with their army of talent. Craig Venter, Francis Collins, and the ever-expanding collections of scientists in their communities were now joining the data-mining crowd and adding substantial new thinking to how data could be used to answer the tough questions of the body and living.

To some, the questions raised by our knowledge of the genome are scary.

Assume, as some began to think, that all diseases were preprogrammed into your system. With this reality, knowing you had this or that "bad" gene would define a period of pensive waiting for something horrible to happen. It also begs the question of whether we have any free will or are simply a collection of future reactions, with the script of our genome being the roadmap of our unchanging destiny.

To others in medicine, the genetic revolution was an awakening because it meant our bodies possessed a far more complex code controlling its growth. To this more optimistic discovery group, we could, through clever and carefully constructed research, build ways of intervening to correct problems before they appeared. In other words, shift from a reactive system of health care to a proactive one.

The very definition of proactive includes the sense of being able to control a future event based on current action—and is the optimistic view of knowing the life script of the individual, with the assumption that the individual's life destiny was not already preordained through the genome he inherited at birth; presenting a set of potential pathways: yes; determining the final course of action: no (at least not always). It is this wealth of data problems that serves as the platform for discovery in the emerging era of PHC.

From the movement to electronic medical records (EMR) to the conceptual model of a national health infrastructure, the problem of data organization is being attacked on a number of fronts with a similar long-term goal—to define a system of individual and information-based medicine that provides the highest quality of care and focuses on health along with disease management. The goal: improve the quality of living for all patients.

But first we are going to have to deal with a change in the world of analysis. Figuring out that an individual has a positive credit score is far easier than understanding the predictive relationships between her genome and her long-term health status. We are about to enter an almost infinite world of data.

Dealing with Information Overload

In the nineteenth century, the challenges of understanding the expanse and depth of medical knowledge was at least manageable by the more clever professionals. The reality of that earlier century was that the amount of knowledge required to do your job as a medical professional was limited—and most competent physicians could (with some work) understand the complete expanse of medicine.

A single physician could know it all.

Another stark reality: solving a patient's problems in the nineteenth century was largely an art, with a smattering of scientific knowledge injected into the mix. Still, science itself was by no means the primary ingredient—or at least science supported by knowledge with certain predictive qualities supporting it.

Now, think back just a decade ago and reconsider the problem.

Ten years ago the medical community experienced an explosion in the areas of diagnostic solutions, had gained depth in their knowledge of the genome, and generally understood the potential of disease and new ways of challenging it. Society had moved from a period where the available knowledge in the field outpaced what the average person could understand.

The range of human capacity, at least as we know how to use it today, shows little disparity between the least and the best of us on this problem. Eventually, nearly everyone experiences data overload, which our emerging world of information has ensured is more than simply a mere possibility.

The change from their colleagues in the nineteenth century was thus dramatic. Where nineteenth-century physicians could easily be the all-knowing experts, their twentieth-century counterparts could not. One physician could not know it all—and the problem of managing data was about to get worse.

Remember the description of HGP and the large number of data points surrounding each of our genetic maps? What I did not highlight was that each of the genes bears a relationship to a larger number of proteins and that these in turn relate back to almost all of the elements of how our bodies operate—including disease and health states. Couple this complex set of data points with the understanding that our genes evolve based on inputs of transcription factors—the various proteins that turn our genes on or off—that cause changes (creating other proteins, causing disease, etc.), and you (and your physician) are suddenly overloaded yet again.

While this land of confusion is turning each of us into the proverbial "deer in the headlights," to the emerging world of data miners this confusion is where the problem becomes interesting. How do you parse through and understand this seemingly infinite set of possibilities?

The answer is with patience, smart algorithms, and computers—and a new breed of really creative scientists.

An Industry of Assessments

Dr. Doreen Robinson and Dr. Paul Schaudies are classic examples of the emerging deep data miners. Operating largely outside of the media glare, they focused on one of the more fascinating issues of data searching and information pattern matching—the ability to use the genetic fingerprint of a known biological molecule to instantly identify it through comparisons with a comprehensive data library. While the HGP was clearly a seminal event in human history, it was only the beginning of what would be an incredibly long journey of discovery with our need to move this knowledge of a basic human vocabulary into a series of short stories on almost all the elements of life that surround us. Robinson and Schaudies decided to attack a different aspect of this vocabulary problem—the identity of specific molecules pertinent to the treatment of disease, including bacteria. They have chosen a problem that has substantial and long-term potential for anyone worried about how infections can kill us.

Most people who grew up in a hospital environment understand the seriousness of infections. The fear that we will one day be facing a host of infectious agents outside our scope of treatments is the ultimate nightmare of the research community, with the increasing "foot race" between the evolution of bacteria and our ability to provide a suitable attack strategy being among the great intellectual tests of our time.

One of the more critical issues for researchers studying infections is in how to rapidly identify the specific infectious agent, defining it at a genetic level and then providing a targeted therapy specifically designed to beat it. Their development issue is in how to define the vocabulary of these genetic fingerprints, store them on the appropriate media, and, finally, correlate the knowledge of that genetic data with an actual physical sample. This is where Robinson and Schaudies became incredibly clever.

Their solution was simple enough, although it involved an extension in knowledge management with as much power as Google. Robinson and Schaudies considered the issue of how to construct dictionaries of genetic fingerprints—and specifically those that would be important in the identification of infectious and other biological agents—as well as how to ensure the dictionary was being incorporated within a patient's testing and treatment cycle.

What is the medical significance of this discovery? Simple. It could save lives.

Speed to treatment is one of the most critical measures of success when attacking severe infections. If too much time passes, the patient may die simply because the bacteria will have spread faster than the patient's body could manage it. Robinson and Schaudies focused on the integration of a data dictionary for infectious agents and its real-time use within clinical environments to ensure that when one of these nastier by-products of our evolution appears in the future, the clinical team will have the ability to instantly identify its type and attack with a targeted treatment. It is ultimately a complex problem of pattern matching and discovery that requires newer technologies and deep data mining.

But not all problems of assessment need to be as complicated. The medical staff at a hospital in the Midwest have demonstrated how even simple data points can define critical conclusions.

Data to Action

Dr. Lee Goldman and the medical team at Cook County Hospital had a problem.

The management of cardiac events represents one of the most time-sensitive problems confronting a physician. Wait too long and the patient can die. Come up with the wrong recommendation and the patient can die. It is a complex problem that requires a mixture of great intuition and clinical data to answer.

But Goldman had an idea. Why not develop a decision tree based on a collection of what he believed were relevant patient observations to rapidly assess the health status of the patient—and determine if they were about to have a heart attack without using the more complex and time-consuming procedures of the day?

So how did he test his hypothesis? He did it the way any outstanding researcher would—he established his protocols, defined test populations, and performed a study. Before we look at the end of this story, let's take a look at a few of the data points he used for his test. The factors were simple.

- Is the patient's electrocardiogram (EKG) normal?
- Is the patient having unstable angina?
- Is there fluid in the patient's lungs?
- Is the patient's systolic blood pressure below 100?

After several years of data collection, the results were in and clear in their conclusions. Goldman's approach was substantially better than the old method of recognizing patients who weren't having a heart attack—the average doctor would guess accurately in between 70 to 89 percent of the cases. Using his algorithm the success rate jumped to 95 percent.[1]

Goldman had, in this case, performed a logical connection of data points in the environment of the patient to draw a conclusion. And when this simple collection of correlations was used by the average physician it was as effective in diagnosis as a trained cardiologist.

Remember the earlier discussion on the expanding array of data points around you and your life equation? Goldman had intuitively used that line of thinking to identify the right collection of connected points to determine a likely outcome. Recognizing that finding the state of perfect "truth" in medicine is an inexact science, he used another of the lessons we use in almost all areas of life—confidence scores.

To be fair to your family doctor, the idea of assessments is not new to the medical community. Were you to enter any physician's office for a first visit, he would likely subject you to a battery of questions concerning your health history and diseases. In this case, the physician is building an information file on what are traditionally viewed as the key data points related to a patient's health status. Physicians may also ask a number of questions related to basic preventive areas, such as immunizations and health habits, in an attempt to predict if you are at risk for developing conditions known to be preventable by the health care community.

These physicians are, like Goldman, helping you better understand the best ways of managing your health or confronting disease. How is this changing in the new era of anywhere/anytime information?

Let's say you're concerned you may have high cholesterol. Today, likely the first place you turned for help is the Internet. However, the Internet is only one source—and probably the only one that does not link the various elements of your personal medical record. Remember, the Internet may be great for getting data that in the old days was available only in a library or printed in a magazine or newspaper, but it falls woefully short when you need to be able to perform a deeper dive within the health information collected by the various members of your health team.

Goldman, your physicians, and the other broader community of health care professionals that provide you with help are building information (and conclusions) on you that you can bet are not showing up in your Internet search on the relevance of HDL and LDL values.

But that problem could change, or at least the limitations of how we search for relevant information. Imagine the world envisioned by complex data miners—nearly infinite collections of data amassed through networks of grid-style processing and storage environments linking everything from your personal health goals to your latest imaging study, the results of every lab test ever performed on you, as well as a recordation of your responses to treatments for a viral infection when you were ten.

The point of this example is that when the various data resources of the health system eventually intertwine with a more global health infrastructure, society will have the ability to create data linkages and develop new forms of knowledge based on a different form of an Internet-type network. The new system of personalized health assessments will have its value multiplied when it becomes a standard part of your interactions with your new health team.

The impact for us as patients is that we will finally be receiving information germane to our unique health condition—not simply the one-size-fits-all advice of the past. But it will, unfortunately, require a substantial amount of work to get there.

The complex alignment of resources that will be required to build our health "currency" or even to construct our future health "ATM-style" network will require the cooperation of a set of larger groups, such as the government, employers, and physicians and health professionals. No matter their loyalty, all groups share at least one common need—the ability to gather and interpret a complex array of data points.

Before we start looking at the larger issues of how all of the pieces will fit together, let's take a look at some of the future "appliances." They are being developed by an industry with a short but interesting set of accomplishments.

Note

1. Lee Goldman, "Multifactorial index of cardiac risk in noncardiac surgical procedures," *New England Journal of Medicine*, October 20, 1977. Malcom Gladwell, *Blink: The Power of Thinking without Thinking* (Little, Brown & Company, 2005).

PART III

CO-REVOLUTIONS

Never trust a computer you can't throw out a window.

—STEVE WOZNIAK

IN 1969, BUSICOM, a small Japanese calculator company, was searching for ways of improving the power of the technology housed within its calculating machines. The calculator market was a competitive place at the time—with the industry focused on finding new and clever ways of making the machines smaller and portable—and Busicom felt it needed some outside help.

In 1969, information technology was definitely not the buzz of the period that it is today. The hot topics were the war in Vietnam, outer space, the creep of communism, and how U.S. cities were being destroyed by the divisive forces of racism and poverty. Luckily for the coming personalized health care (PHC) revolution, a number of innovators in our engineering community had their eyes on other problems—with the issue of how to take advantage of the emerging power of the semiconductor at the top of the list. One of the first to feel the potential of this revolution was the calculator—the then ubiquitous symbol of technological prowess.

In 1970, and in what proved to be a seismic event in the market, the Sharp Corporation introduced the first handheld, battery-powered calculator. Suddenly the technology race was on—rendering those who did not react fast enough, or with the right marketing savvy, destined for the graveyard.

And Busicom thought that it was ready for the chase.

A year before Sharp's historic announcement, Busicom had approached Intel about its development problem, which turned out to be a seminal time in history, and for reasons that almost no one at the time understood. The microcomputer was about to be born, and as history later recounted, it was largely an accident.

The 1969-era Intel was a small, technically skilled developer of memory chips. Although it was nowhere near the household name it is today, Busicom's selection of the Intel band of engineers was nonetheless a logical choice.

Busicom understood that the soon-to-be-developed microprocessor would be critical to propel its calculator ahead in the competitive world of consumer electronics. It also appreciated that Intel had the right combination of smarts and drive to help it pull it off. While Intel was recognized for its experience in building electronics products, it was also known by the reputation of one of its founders, Robert Noyce. Noyce had been a leading figure in the development of the integrated circuit and considered a pioneer in the emerging computer electronics industry.

The Busicom and Intel alliance started one of the major threads of change that would become a cornerstone of the future practices of PHC—the rise of microprocessor and microcontroller-based products. The applications and evolutions since the 1969 birth of the Intel microprocessor have been staggering.

My focus in part III is on the growth of one of the most powerful enablers of PHC—the unique capabilities of the microcomputer and digital storage to manage data and extend our decision-making process. The chapters in this section will explore the evolving set of data and knowledge utilities being defined by the computer industry and discuss how they are theoretically and practically enhancing our abilities to manage the expanding world of data. The fundamental concept behind this new computer architecture is the creation of what I call the human/machine partnership. And it starts with a basic fact: we clearly have access to lots of data.

One of the driving challenges facing society in the post Internet world is our knowledge explosion and our inability to manage it—or the "knowledge paradox." If nothing else, the Internet has demonstrated that the world is becoming a sea of data points, often confusing, sometimes important, but always growing. How can we expect to manage this complexity?

A relevant example in medicine is the question of what causes the transformations from normal cell to abnormal in cancer and how these changes are linked back to the genetic blueprint of the individual. Is it a marker (or gene) that was present at birth? Is it the result of some external impact (e.g., X-rays or exposure to a toxin)? The possibilities quickly blend to a confusing picture of alternatives.

In the end, the knowledge paradox establishes a challenge for us in how to construct utilities for parsing through and then incorporating the expanding complexity of our world into our actions. Would we, for example, knowingly take Vioxx if we understood that it, in combination with our internal biology, had the potential to cause heart failure? Would we have taken that extra dose of Tylenol when we had the flu knowing that it could lead to liver failure? The goal of these knowledge utilities is to prevent that from happening. But how do you move from this set of ideas to the finished product?

I believe the answer will start with the computer—and how we learn to connect with its vast potential.

To understand the ways this human/machine architecture can address the problems of information overload I will divide the emerging "computer" solutions into two distinct components: the combination of human intellect with a machine (the human/machine model) and the use of a machine in isolation to read, interpret, and act (the machine/machine model). Both of these machine architectures are examples of a new form of information utility enabled by the intersection of the computer, information, and communication industries. It is this collection of technologies that I will weave throughout the final chapter as examples of the types of thinking we will use to build our new systems of PHC.

Remember the story *2001: A Space Odyssey* (1968) and the demented computer HAL? The power and danger of HAL was that it clearly had the "intelligence" to run the life-support systems of the spaceship, but also lacked the insights of what we would expect in a compassionate fellow traveler. The machine in the story had a set of rules, it was going to operate by them, and the humans that lived within its environments would be forced to accept the outcome—even if that meant death. HAL, as the futurist's worst nightmare, was the overly intelligent machine taking control of the world. And more important, HAL was an example of the ultimate machine/machine model. It could think—that is, it had some form of internal intelligence—it could understand its environment, and it could perform actions.

But our future world of machine/machine solutions does not have to go to that extreme—and has potential value that is incalculable. The insulin pump, which connects a real-time, machine-based measurement of blood glucose with a machine-driven insulin-delivery vehicle, is an example of this type of future application and represents a major improvement for the diabetes community. And the good news is that absolutely no one would confuse the insulin pump with HAL—its various users tend to really like it.

Yes, the pancreas is still the world's best way to monitor and control the distribution of insulin in our bodies. But a machine that does the same thing is nice to have—and substantially better than the constant finger pricking and injections that are the daily experiences of a diabetic. Yet it has some glaring limitations.

While the insulin pump can measure the level of insulin within certain areas of our bodies—that is, traveling through our blood vessels—our pancreas as part of a larger system is working with information coming from a potential trillion sources. And our pancreas has the ability to react to and perform subtle changes that our crude measurements of glucose and the insulin pump lack the power to understand. We have an endless expanse of discovery ahead of us, with the more we find out showing us how much more we need to understand.

So where will we go next? Interestingly, the answer begins in the world of the binary.

A Digital World

What does "being digital" actually mean? On one level, digital is simply the vocabulary underpinning our computers and an engineering offshoot of the base 2 field of math.

If you were to tear inside the guts and hardware of a computer device, you would be confronted with a single elegant building block, the binary world of zeros and ones. While it may be difficult to understand, a computer uses this basic alphabet as its foundation for solving absolutely every problem it faces. Storing your photographs, a book, the music from your iPod, or an e-mail message all rely on this fundamental vocabulary.

In the pre-electronic era, knowledge was often the gold of professions, with the ability of knowledge workers (e.g., doctors and lawyers) to define, manage, and generally control the information of their industries—allowing them to maintain a mystique and separateness in society. The computer has altered this world, with a corresponding change for a large number of professionals. Knowledge has evolved to a different state, with the Internet only emphasizing how portable it can become and how instantly it can evolve.

Computers are also challenging our physical borders.

In the precomputer era, the general definition of community was straightforward. People described their communities as the place where they lived. The computer and the Internet have combined to challenge this reality in ways far beyond the telephone and automobiles (two groundbreaking achievements on their own) by providing alternative ways of building our collection of colleagues outside of where we live and across the globe based on interests—not simply location.

The final and one of the most exciting co-revolutions is in the area of artificial intelligence (AI). The underlying theme of AI is that the processing power of the computer (often times coupled with robust communications technologies) has the potential to address increasingly more complex problems that we thought were limited to human ingenuity.

How will these future machines get their power to understand us? The answer will be constructed largely on the platform of our human map. It is this data/information/knowledge transformation defined by our human maps that will ultimately establish our new family of human/machine hybrids. So how are we going to start attacking them? Google has shown us a few obvious ways.

It starts with Web searching.

CHAPTER 7

INFORMATION TO KNOWLEDGE

G OOGLE IS A wonderful example of how fast the world of information has evolved since the movement went digital, with almost every element of media being transformed and made available online. More than being a great way of searching through the Internet, Google also signifies the robustness of the information industry and how the world and definition of data is expanding. Consider how quickly the market has evolved.

Today more than 1.1 billion of our global population of 6.4 billion is connected to the Internet. And since its initial public offering (IPO) in August 2004, the market cap of Google has grown to over $223 billion (December 2007). The world is spinning faster, or at least it seems that way. If you have any doubts about the speed of change, ask anyone who uses the Internet to buy airline tickets, sell products, or search for health information. Our planet has become one big set of connections, with tools like Google becoming the new version of what the librarian used to be—the first place we go when we need a general set of pointers on our quest for information—and the Internet as the world's new community and marketplace.

And it could not have come at a better time.

A 2003 study from the University of California at Berkeley tracked the annual amount of new information being generated by the global community of information brokers. The number it quoted coming from all of the world's media sources is staggering. According to the Berkeley study[1], our global population added roughly five exabytes of new information to the planet's information warehouse in the year 2002 (or 5,000,000,000,000,000,000 bytes). To put that into a different context, that amount of information is the equivalent of having each person on the planet adding about 800 megabytes (MB) of new data to their "personal" hard disks (assuming a world population of 6.3 billion) each year. For those more accustomed to thinking about storage in terms of paper and printed materials, this would be equivalent to roughly thirty feet of printed paper. That same Berkeley study also revealed that five exabytes of information is equivalent to roughly 250,000 trees worth of printed materials.

This does not account for the impact of the exploding information that our research on the genome is about to unleash on our world. We had better start thinking about how we are going to define and manage the value of this data.

A Different Currency

Prior to the revolutions in computer storage, the way people managed data was relatively simple. If you needed to collect information, you created a paper-based file, put it in a storage cabinet, and searched for it when it was needed.

In 1907, Henry Plummer, a physician at the Mayo Clinic, designed one of the earliest information management solutions in medicine. He created the industry's first medical record, which was to later emerge as a critical element of the future data-management architecture in health care. In the Plummer system all clinic visits and hospital stays were stored in a single file, traveling with the patient as they moved from one unit of the hospital to another.

Today when you want to gather information on a topic, individual, or whatever, not only can you find it in almost any format (print, sound, image, or video), it's likely most of it can be delivered electronically and instantly. And chances are that your search will be through the Internet, with a tool like Google becoming your roadmap. While we may not have had organized sources of information available to us—medical or otherwise—in the days preceding the Plummer invention, we definitely do today.

But how would you like to have all of the information on absolutely every transaction you made, every illness you had, and every job you took appear in someone else's database and then having that person (or company) build recommendations on you that impact your future? Sound scary? It should and it is already happening—consider how it works.

The next time you make a purchase at the grocery store and use your credit card or store loyalty program, chances are good that information about you is being logged into a system that will eventually be used by a variety of players to decipher everything from your buying preferences to your credit worthiness. From the concepts of credit scoring to driving records, the use of information and decision-support models have not only permeated our lives, they have transformed the way we work, think about purchases, and are evaluated. One of the most powerful companies working in this new field of data analytics is the Fair Isaac Corporation—probably a name that you have never heard of before.

A fundamental problem for the credit industry has been how to determine which individuals among their many applicants would most likely repay a loan and who would not. Taking on customers who fail to meet the obligations of a contract is a mess for everyone involved—with the threats of litigation introducing a number of issues for the company that issued the credit card and the person who caused the problem in the first place. Fair Isaac had some ideas on how to solve the problem.

Fair Isaac has taken the questions of data management and demonstrated how data becomes information, turning into a new type of "knowledge" currency. The Fair Isaac value in the credit process has tremendous parallels to what will be required in the health care industry—the need for a system to determine the "knowledge" elements hidden in the vast repositories of data. In the case of the credit industry, whether a collection of diverse data points could define the credit worthiness of an individual is not a question, it's a fact. In contrast to the issues facing the credit-reporting industry, figure 7.1 demonstrates the unique data-mining complexity con-

Figure 7.1. Moving from Randomness to Outcomes

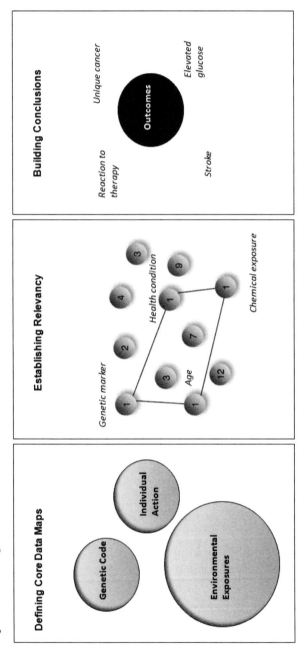

fronting health care, where even defining truth and certainty is tough. From the start of a vast sea of data observations taken from our genome, environment, and actions, we must establish relevancy—the relationships of interconnected variables—and finally define outcomes.

And we must do this all within the confines of a noisy and confusing world of observations. It is an extremely difficult task.

This collection of data-mapping issues is the major question facing society as we move to a system of health information "currency." But, for Fair Isaacs and the financial world, the problem is relatively easy to understand.

Obtaining a credit history on an individual is a data-mining problem involving things like payment amounts and dates. The truth and accuracy of this information is generally easy to prove, although credit reports are not without their mistakes. But how will we build this set of information resources for the health care industry and hope to create the type of analytical framework that Fair Isaacs has excelled in building?

It is this need for complexity that confronts even the most creative among us as we examine the issues of health care data management. Just a few years ago it would have been highly unusual, for example, for a department of radiology to bundle its online image system (assuming, of course, that it even had one) with the larger patient repositories housed in a hospital. Now add to this that the radiology department is only one of the many places the patient encounters in her movement through the health system and you get an idea of just how complex the problem has become. And what about the local environment in which the patient lives? Is there a "Love Canal" in his neighborhood that we do not yet know about—or does she have some combination of genes that modifies her reactions in ways that we do not understand?

And how do we move from simply having information (albeit information that is not yet complete) to having the ability to act on it?

We really need some help.

The Autonomic Engine

So how are we going to manage this explosive growth of information required to build our systems of PHC? Luckily for us, the converging revolutions of computer technology are occurring in parallel with our growth of basic science knowledge—and are providing us with an additional set of tools to solve the problem.

The ultimate answer, I believe, parallels the organization of how our brains process information—or what I call the autonomic and the directed machines. The difference in how these two knowledge utilities (or human/machine hybrids) will process information is critical to understand because they represent the distinct approaches for managing the data overload problem ahead of us. They also represent applications that are already appearing and enable, among other things, the work described earlier of Robinson and Schaudies as they use computer technology to discover the identity of a pathogen and the elegant blend of a machine and our bodies in the insulin pump.

What is the potential of this human and machine combination and how will we realize it? We need to first understand the elements of the new computer platforms, which, like our bodies, come with their own sets of unique potential and complexity. The place to start is the rise of "personal" computing.

The breakout event of the personal computer was arguable when IBM entered the consumer market for computers in the early 1980s. The IBM personal computer and the Microsoft operating system helped to establish the new vocabulary of our era with the concepts of hard drive storage (and now USB keys), graphical user interfaces, and finally the electronic office becoming part of the common vernacular. Who has not heard of Microsoft Word, Excel, and PowerPoint? Practically no one.

The personal computer (along with its offshoot, the microcontroller) has come to represent the reference framework for the "body" in the new era of machine intelligence. They house the core components—processing engine, memory, storage, applications, and communications—that will be used to define this new generation of information utility.

What's next? The answer to this question is where this co-revolution becomes interesting. The reach of computing power is today positioned to move well beyond physical walls—and has the potential to enter our world through a variety of connection points. Along with showing us how to publish and share information, the computer is providing us with ever more clever ways of socializing, including through the use of chat rooms, e-mail, and a variety of evolving and more creative ways of engaging in dialogs.

But there is more to the story. The computer is now beginning to move beyond its physically constrained existence—its early limitations of being trapped within the confines of its computer casing, keyboard, and screen—and starting to get information on you and your environment and acting on it. How does this happen? Easy: through sensors.

The growth of sensor technologies is one of the more fascinating evolutions of our digital world. Providing the ability to detect action (like temperature) and observation (like video), they have introduced a set of "eyes and ears" to our computer platforms—extending their reach beyond the screen and mouse that we normally associate with as their input and output controls. What does this mean for PHC? The growth of remote-sensor technologies has dramatically extended the ability of the computer to engage in support of our bodies and movements within our world. And it is happening around you in ways that you are probably not even thinking about.

As you read the pages of this book your brain is controlling a number of your body's higher-level functions without your guidance—for example, your heart beating. These activities are being managed as part of a broader collection of systems and according to a balance that is required to sustain your life and well understood by your brain. Your body effectively has a set of rules of operations that it uses to manage these various systems and ensures that they are performed accurately and as part of some master blueprint—and it does so largely outside of your thinking or control.

The autonomic engine operates according to a similar principle, with the combination of logic rules and sensors allowing these packaged applications to operate without requiring any human direction. Yes, they will be acquiring information either from you or your environment, but no, they will not require you to tell them how to operate. Anyone walking around with a pacemaker understands how this type of product works.

In contrast the directed engine requires that you act on its messages to complete it tasks. Although it may also include the ability to act on information that it senses within your body and manage this information according to a set of rules and its own logic controller, the directed engine ultimately requires that you, the human, provide the final control. But the end product is the same: these new forms of human/machine and machine/machine models will be extending our ability to manage the complexity of our worlds far beyond what we can solely using our individual human capacity.

The good news is that these new knowledge utilities are already being used by most of us today—at least those of us who use the Internet and tools like Google. While it may not seem obvious, Google and the other search engines represent one of the early examples of machine-based solutions for managing information overload. Imagine trying to move through the nearly infinite collection of nodes on the Internet to search for relevant information on a question. The software algorithms of Google manage that problem for you.

So while the tasks and accomplishments of Google may appear simple (i.e., the general concept of parsing through data to match a question to an answer), they represent one of the seminal building blocks to the larger challenges facing our movement to machine-based intelligence. The vitality of Google is showing just how far we have moved and how we now have the basic tools to transform unconnected and incoherent data to knowledge.

Before we dive into the weeds of what this new family of knowledge utilities will look for, it is time to meet a new set of neighbors and the second major revolution of the computer industry—the growth of the virtual—and see how it is starting to impact health care.

Note

1. "How Much Information?" University of California at Berkeley, School of Information Management and Systems, 2003.

CHAPTER 8

VIRTUAL COMMUNITIES

I N 1993, HOWARD RHEINGOLD, a noted technology futurist, led a dialogue on the vast changes of the post-Internet
world.[1] His theory was simple. The border-breaking expanse of
our global communications network had provided a way for individuals to find others with similar interests and to begin an orderly set
of information exchanges based on the emerging tools available in
the now "virtual" world. We had moved from the earth as a place
defined by land and space, to a world of connections defined by elec-
tricity and content.

Now enter the era of the Internet in our post–twentieth-century
world.

As Rheingold predicted, we have added multiple layers of meaning to the term "community," enhancing our ability to establish its
border through qualities other than location. You can, for example,
just as easily label yourself a member of a community whose members live down the street from you as on the other side of the planet.
And as Web sites like MySpace and Facebook have clearly demonstrated, the Internet has led to an explosion of virtual connections,
with the requirements for membership no longer based on location.

This concept and growth of the virtual is a critical element of the
move to personalized health care (PHC)—and it will be supported
by a number of organizational parameters. Among them is the notion
that the virtual community can be governed by an evolving set of
laws, many of which would be borrowed in whole or in part from
their "physical" counterparts—including systems of exchange.

Another major theme is the ability to adapt to and manage change. The virtual community would have the ability to redefine its rules and regulations on the fly, if needed. Consider the impact of complex media on these emerging social organizations.

In the pre-broadband era of the Internet, the movement of large data files like video clips was nearly impossible. Drinking through a small straw of your telephone line would only allow so much flow of information—the original dial-up modems were limited to a speed of roughly 56kps. Today (less than a decade and a millennium of change later) is vastly different, with most people having at least access to a cable provider and a high-speed link and Web sites such as YouTube that demonstrate the power of video to communicate ideas.

Is this global and borderless future inevitable? The facts are supporting Rheingold's vision and also showing us that this new form of Internet community can be used in a positive way—including improving almost all elements of society, with health care being one of the major beneficiaries.

So when will the revolution in health care begin? The good news is that it has already started, with the growth of virtual communities now being institutionalized through a large number of patient support groups and even the professional practices of medicine. One of the more interesting developments has been within a group of professionals that you would have probably assumed were as far away from a computer keyboard as anyone in medicine: the world's community of cardiac surgeons.

CTSNet: Building Community in Medicine

One of the most powerful examples of building a virtual community is the work of Drs. Bob Replogle, Peter Greene, and their colleagues on CTSNet. With the Internet as its community platform, CTSNet has broken down the previous borders of country and created a unified and virtual whole linking the world's cardiac surgeons within the virtual space of the Internet's communication pipes. Following the lead of the Internet and its ability to redefine the definition and location of workplace, it has done so without having a large corporate location supporting its growth. With a small support team operating out of waterfront office in downtown Baltimore, CTSNet could just have easily established itself in rural Alaska. The "offices" and "products" of CTSNet are, in the end, the workspace of the Internet.

And there is another great innovation—real-time knowledge distribution. Not too many people read last week's news. We take for granted the ability of the daily paper to capture the most current thinking in our society and to provide that to us via its printed (and now electronic) pages. CTSNet and the other emerging virtual communities operate with the new paradigm of knowledge distribution, which means that knowledge has now become an immediate currency that is available practically everywhere and in different forms. Would you like to get your information on your phone or iPod—or would you prefer reading it on your PC? Knowledge, which could easily become stale in the predigital world, can be dynamically updated in these now-virtual communities and take advantage of the new form of knowledge currency that I highlighted earlier.

How would you like your cardiac surgeon operating on you using a technique that had been demonstrated as ineffective or worse, dangerous, in the broader community of surgery? With CTSNet this notion of "stale" ideas can at least be instantly challenged at Internet speed making sure that your surgeon knows what works and does not before they start cutting into your chest.

Greene, Replogle, and their colleagues on CTSNet are part of an information movement in medicine and helping to build a future of real time, connected and accepted knowledge. What else is happening with these emerging virtual communities? The next set of changes is as old as society—commerce—but this time with a new set of tools.

Buying and Selling

The world of selling has largely remained the same since we first figured out that we could get something from someone else by exchanging one good for another. In the pre-money era, these exchanges occurred through an elaborate bartering system. You trade a pig for five chickens. You might not eat any bacon but you'll enjoy many mornings of scrambled eggs.

With the introduction of currency, the notion of the even exchange became easier. Instead of relying on the art of negotiation to define value on various objects, the government did the hard part by assigning a value to the money (say, gold) a buyer and seller used to complete a transaction. A number of innovations and refinements have occurred in the financial world along the way, with the most obvious being the idea that money, while measured as an accumulation of value, may not physically have to be exchanged between the parties as long as at some point in time a reconciliation could be performed, including through checks, credit cards, and wire transfers.

But to really get a sense for how the old rules of the physical are being integrated in our new electronic communities it is time to say hello and thanks to Jeff Bezos and his incredible perseverance. While not the first, Bezos and his colleagues are helping to redefine one of the most basic forms of commerce in our society—the store and its customers.

Jeff Bezos and the investors behind Amazon had a vision of how the globally connected Internet could be used for redefining the interactions of a purchaser and supplier. It was an approach that builds upon the tried-and-true model of having goods for sale and a retail site in which to sell them. Where we once relied on the physical store (aka, the "brick and mortar"), Bezos pushed that concept into the virtual and brought the physical store into your home—albeit one in which you could not touch the goods or immediately take them home with you.

But Bezos and his team were addressing only one form of commerce—that involving organizations (stores) and individuals (customers). What about the interactions that we have with one another, where we are trying to sell something that we own to another person (and not a store)—and are attempting to get the best possible price? This is where the founders of eBay introduced us to yet another form of commerce: the online auction.

The neighborhood flea market had just entered the twenty-first century with the result that absolutely everyone could become their own version of an Amazon store—but this time built around basic bargaining as the way of setting the price.

eBay established an exchange between the seller and purchaser—allowing the market to determine interests and prices through an "electronic" auction—and transferred the responsibility of who would maintain the inventory away from the virtual store (the Bezos model) to the person who actually possessed the product. And unlike the old-style model of stores and inventories, eBay became a broad environment in which the use of the Internet for the exchange of goods was the value proposition.

This eBay extension in thinking is critical because it highlights another use of the knowledge economies infrastructure—the ability to use the Internet and the virtual world as the destination and link between the user/customer and the provider of the goods or service. The value is no longer the "bricks and mortar," it is the pipeline or transaction environment. And in the case of the Internet, this pipeline can exist anywhere and act anytime. The impacts of these commerce exchanges on health care are potentially enormous.

Using this eBay model you can imagine a world in which each of your information and product requests are handled via a broker whose mission in life is to manage one aspect of the health care supply chain—providing you with multiple sourcing options and helping to establish the lowest price. What would it be like, for example, if you could enter an online community and search through a variety of suppliers for the medication you required—and allow the market to drive the best price? It would probably be better than the system of fixed pricing and contracts we face today.

And guess what? It is already starting to happen in subtle ways around you, with our colleagues in radiology demonstrating how easily the Internet can be used to service a patient's complex health needs.

Building a Health Care Exchange

The recent and fast growth of the Nighthawk Radiology Corporation is a little known example of a technology platform to manage the professional needs of a customer community—and an excellent introduction to the future systems of brokered health care. While a favorite of the financial community, few outside of the company founders probably recognize the Nighthawk value in reshaping the paradigm of medicine.

Their premise is a simple one. Using the Web-based Nighthawk information network, a patient (through their local physician) can gain access to a specialist radiologist with absolutely no consideration of location. Nighthawk becomes the equivalent of the modern marketplace, with the various buyers and sellers using the Internet as their only form of linkage. Nighthawk provides the professional talent (the radiologists) and the transaction network, and buyers contract for their services through the virtual community of the Internet. There is no storefront and no single dedicated imaging center. And the Nighthawk network is infinitely reconfigurable and can grow (and retract) simply based on the needs of the customers in its eBay-style marketplace.

Will the health care system eventually embrace the broader pricing models of the eBay model and move to dynamic pricing based on availability and demand? The answer is yes, with Nighthawk and CTSNet showing how this can be done in health care. The parallels to eBay to Nighthawk are straightforward.

Although not as rapidly changing as the second-by-second bidding experiences of eBay, Nighthawk allows the various buyers and sellers to engage in a form of price negotiation. The "actors" in the Nighthawk system must agree and live with price and delivery rules as they engage in professional services to support the needs of a patient case. CTSNet attacks a different, although equally important, issue of these newer commerce environments—the need to define users, profiles, and ways of communicating. In the ether of CTSNet you become a member, have a profile, and can interact with other members of the virtual community with your identity defined by this now online profile. In this virtual space of CTSNet your identity is purely defined by what you have within the profile of the many pages of the CTSNet web. And it builds upon the same ideas pioneered by eBay and underscored by MySpace and the various social networking web sites—the concept of electronic identity. Consider, for example, the maturing rules in eBay.

In order to enter into the eBay world of commerce, you must become a member. As you become more involved, whether you're a buyer, seller, or both, you accrue a rating based on how well you played according to the rules of the eBay road.

For example, if you're a deadbeat, meaning you won an auction but failed to pay for an item as agreed, the seller has the right to assign negative feedback to your membership account. While not a requirement, individuals have the option to comment on other individuals they connect with in the eBay community—and have those comments appear on the individual's "personalized" record. Similar to our example of the credit-scoring industry, a new form of evaluation has been created that will travel around with this individual in the virtual community of eBay.

You are building a new profile on "who you are"—and a potentially alternate ego to the one known by your friends and neighbors. You may be known as quiet and unassuming at work, but within these new virtual community models you can become almost any type of character you can imagine or would really like to be.

Along with the concept of data capture and record keeping, the eBay world has also established a set of operating parameters and supports the concepts of unique functional identity. You can enter the eBay universe simply as someone interested in finding a particular good or service, bidding on it, and, if the highest bidder, buying it. You can also enter eBay as someone selling an item (or items) and use eBay as a virtual storefront with some limits. But you cannot, for example, use eBay to sell your kidneys[2]—which someone tried—or engage in illegal activities.

But that's not all. Along with the various system "actors," the presence of eBay has led to a class of information utilities that exist only within the space of the Internet and are allowing us to give birth to new forms of computer life. One of the most notable of these new life forms is PayPal.

What is PayPal? PayPal has emerged as one of the leading ways of entering into a commercial exchange on the Internet (paying for a product) with another individual and/or company. Rather than paying for a purchase directly from a bank account, say, using a debit card or sending money via the mail somehow, the PayPal model is based on the premise a buyer would prefer to have someone act as their broker in the virtual and untouchable world of the Internet—ensuring the seller received their payment while protecting you in the case of fraud.

You could easily argue that this is exactly what the VISA system does today in regular commerce—and could easily do in the virtual world. And you would be right, at least partially. The beauty of the PayPal model is that it is a system of financial exchange totally built around the power and thinking of the Internet and the digital world while carrying absolutely no legacy issues from the "old" VISA approach. PayPal is an agent and arbitrator for you and has no physical existence other than on the Internet.

Ultimately PayPal and eBay represent striking examples of how a virtual community can build itself, establish and incorporate the concepts of personalization, and, finally, ensure that the community is governed by a set of ethical and practical rules of engagement.

Now let's return to health care and examine another example of how communities are appearing that incorporate these emerging information-driven services—and the product and committed efforts of two physicians from the intensive care unit. Their work demonstrates one of the more interesting examples of a health "market" in action.

The eICU: Redefining Borders

As almost everyone who has entered into a health care exchange understands, the complicated media of the human body often demand a complex information infrastructure. From the use of 3-D modeling tools in cardiology to the data representation issues brought on by the genetics industry, the information management challenges in health care rival the best problems of the engineering world. The industry is facing large data objects, a need for rapid reaction, and, finally, the possibility of causing harm to a patient if an error occurs either in omission or in application. One of the newer and more powerful information utilities in the health field is the market offering defined by Drs. Mike Breslow and Brian Rosenfeld of the VisiCu Corporation.

Managing an intensive care unit (ICU) requires an integration of highly skilled professionals and advanced technology. It is an area of medicine, similar to surgery, that requires an attention to fine details and split-second reactions.

Enter the Breslow and Rosenfeld telemedicine system. Tested within the confines of an academic medical center, the Breslow and Rosenfeld team took the problem of ICU physician monitoring—how to most effectively monitor the complex stream of information surrounding a patient in the ICU environment—as a market opportunity. Recognizing that the advances in communications and computer processing provided a foundation for a dramatically different service model, the VisiCu team constructed one of the world's early remote-monitoring applications for critically ill patients.

But they began their development with a little help—the biggest being that the idea of remote monitoring is not necessarily a new one and happens every day in almost every hospital. Walk into any nurses' station and chances are you will see a number of monitors showing the physical status of the patients housed in that unit. In many ways, this nurses' station has come to represent a local information repository—where various members of the health care team can come to check the status of the patients and exchange ideas.

The ICU is no different. By definition, an ICU patient requires intensive care administered around the clock. This is where the Breslow and Rosenfeld team successfully thought outside of the box. Understanding that physician time is expensive and that the job of the intensive care specialist is challenging—and represents a commodity in short supply in a number of places—the two men had an idea. What if rather than having the remote monitoring of the patients take place down the hall from the patients, the monitoring location was relocated to the home of the physician or some other facility outside of the hospital.

Similar in some ways to the model defined by the Nighthawk Radiology group, the eICU would be constructed on the backbone of a robust and secure information network in which the location of the physician professional was less important than the service being provided. While basic in concept, it represented a revolutionary convergence of a number of approaches that were already in use within security monitoring firms, and the medial equipment industry, with the now ubiquitous delivery of communications and processing. The combined outcome of a more efficient use of physician resources and broader and more effective coverage for patients within the ICU was not only striking in its value proposition, it helped to improve the quality of medical care. And the Breslow and Rosenfeld team had the numbers to prove it.

Although the efforts of the eICU are no doubt important and represent a major forward for the industry, I believe that we are only at the beginning stage of what these virtual communities could provide. Where will these evolving communities go next?

Health as an Open Market

Jeff Bezos believed that the new tools of the digital age would transform how people purchased books and set to rebuild an industry through his company, Amazon. It was a task that would consume years of effort, literally billions of dollars, and a change in how people thought about their book purchases.

Will this same change happen overnight in health care? First, let's ponder the complexity of the problem. Health is ultimately a personal exchange involving an array of choices by individuals within the construct of a well-defined system: when you are sick, you see a doctor. The doctor prescribes a medicine and you visit the pharmacy.

In exploring the commerce engines of the Internet, Bezos and his colleagues attacked specific elements of book distribution and retailing. Their achievements demonstrated how tools of the knowledge economy can be used to help improve the process of existing industries, and in some cases, define new commercial spaces.

Although the system of PHC will benefit from the revolutionary/transformational thinking of Bezos and others, a broader challenge exists. How can society manage and define the almost limitless collection of data elements required on the human machine? And how do we then include this evolving knowledge within an exchange system—or will the complexity of health care require the growth of an ever increasing number of exchange models similar to those we have discussed throughout this chapter? It is an interesting collection of challenges ahead of us.

Some of these emerging communities will no doubt share similarities with eBay and involve the direct human-to-human connection of patient with professionals for help.

Others, like Nighthawk, will emerge linking patient problems with an expanding collection of online professionals—each bringing different views of the problem and hopefully adding to the range of knowledge used to interpret the patient case.

Finally, others will emerge that allow patients and professionals to link within a globally connected supply network in which we begin to establish true "value" for our broader health care system—and building parity in the world's markets. Is it fair, for example, for one country to pay one price for a pharmaceutical and another to be charged a higher rate simply because they did not get the best deal? This final type of market-supply community would take us all a lot closer to a real market economy in health care and eliminate the artificial taxes that many members of society are forced to endure.

The ultimate answer to this exchange question—and the issue of how many types of communities will be created—starts with a basic reality: The information economy and its technical solutions have provided a new set of authoring tools and a way to deliver the information. The question is how to best tap into the vocabulary of the human body while describing it in a way people can understand and use within these emerging exchange models.

But we have another problem ahead of us: the complexity of the actions that take place at the end of the "pipes." Our bodies contain an innumerable collection of intertwined and unique "systems" and require an expanding cast of professionals to help. As I discussed on the mapping problem, the question of depth and orientation is a big one for us—with a need to discover the "root" of a problem through a confusing sea of alternatives.

So what would happen if we took this idea of community and exchange and brought it to the level of how your internal body's chemistry was changing and allowed these changes to be communicated to a different type of community and community intelligence? Could your heart, for example, become a member of its own "community" and maintain a dialog with other interested parties through the information technologies that support CTSNet, the eICU and Nighthawk?

The example of this final and more complex form of exchange systems is already in your neighborhood. But this time it is not coming through your doctor's office or housed within your local hospital. The future of health care can be seen in an unlikely place—your local garage and the various mechanics that service your car.

I know by experience. I have one of the more creative ones living near me.

Notes

1. Howard Rheingold, "Cold Knowledge and Social Warmth." *Newsweek,* September 6, 1993, p. 49.

2. "Online shoppers bid millions for human kidney," CNN/Associated Press, September 3, 1999.

CHAPTER 9

MACHINE-BASED INTELLIGENCE

ANDY PETER runs a small auto-repair shop outside of Annapolis, Maryland.

Over the years, Peter has developed a reputation as an outstanding car mechanic. Although his specialty is foreign-built engines, he is also an expert in sensors and decision-support technologies.

If you recently purchased a car, you have been dragged into the world of sensor technologies. Unlike their predecessors of twenty years back, our current automobiles would not move without the interaction of microprocessors and sophisticated sensors providing data on everything from fuel mixtures to whether your vehicle has been hit by someone. One sign of the times: it has been estimated that today's car contains as much as one hundred meters of wiring.

Why the dramatic change in the industry? A number of factors converged in the auto industry, ranging from issues of emissions to consumer preferences and safety. One example of an industry change agent has been pollution control.

Poorly managed auto emissions are a terrible problem for society. Car exhaust imposes devastating impacts on our quality of life and is also generally harmful to the environment (with global warming being another dangerous outcome). Because automobile manufacturers want you to drive, one way they have responded to this challenging is by installing computers and sensors (the electronic control unit, or ECU) in our vehicles that monitor the efficiency of our cars' engines. The birth of the ECU, which occurred in the 1980s, has given rise to more costly car repair bills if it malfunctions and created a whole new generation of auto mechanics like Peter. He and those gifted with his talents are as facile with a wrench as they are adept in utilizing a computer to determine the health of your car.

The change of Peter's world as a mechanic, and our driving experience, is linked to the revolutions of the information-technology industry. The ever-increasing miniaturization of computer technology and the corresponding increase in processing power has given rise to a wide array of creative ways of thinking about how to incorporate computers into our environments. The car is simply the easiest and most relevant example for people to experience, and it demonstrates the two basic issues related to the value of sensors: the ability to obtain internal (operating within the car) and external (operating around the car) information to influence how your vehicle operates.

So while he quietly works out of his garage office, Peter employs several of the critical concepts of personalization in his practice—including understanding the relevance of unique data values and how to separate the background noise from "truth." Peter and his colleagues in the auto-repair industry are in the vanguard of our emerging industry of human/machine intelligence.

And it all starts with data, which, if we are lucky, will somehow be transformed into useful knowledge.

Redefining Physical Encounters

One way the puzzle pieces can start fitting together is this: we know we have near infinite data available to us. To capitalize on the data explosion, people have created ways of organizing and searching that help establish a sense of order out of the chaos.

Next, the Web community built a set of rules of engagement and defined communities with basic properties to cover simple exchanges between the actors (for example, eBay and CTSNet).

The final test is in how to establish tools to automate the decision-making issues of control—to define our human/machine and machine/machine models and build the autonomic and directed engines.

One of the technological advantages of eBay's virtual community model is that it has the beauty of limiting its world to the physical connections of computers over the Internet. As discussed earlier, our systems of PHC are more complex and will evolve over an unlimited number of playing fields—including the Internet, clinics, the home, work environments, and, finally, the increasing complexity and depth of the human body.

Our delivery models of PHC will thus force us to begin thinking of new ways of connecting the patient to their health condition and effectively moving the decision-support model to an almost anywhere/anytime model.

How will this be accomplished? One of the more clever examples of this future machine support system was designed by Dr. Dadong Wan. And like a number of other great people in the science community his name is probably unknown to you.

In the late 1990s, Wan was a senior scientist in Accenture's corporate research lab in Chicago, Illinois. Among other things, Wan spent his days thinking about the issues of how to track and manage information within a patient's home. He has invented a near boundless set of ideas that reinvent the ways we interact with information—and the issues facing his research are substantial.

Given the incessant flow of information around us and the often confusing pictures it paints, it is difficult when we are not at full capacity to do everything we are supposed to, when we are supposed to do it. As we all understand, life is filled with various up and down moments and we are not always operating in peak form, which becomes an increasing issue for us as we age and confront an array of deteriorating body systems.

Consider the problem of coping with life confronting an elderly parent.

You might wonder what your elderly parents are doing when you're not there to help and support them. Are they remembering to take their medications, turn off the oven, and blow out the candle they lit? Or what happens if they fall and can't move—how will they seek help? In almost every example we can imagine, some kind of sensor (i.e., video cameras, sound recorders, motion detectors, etc.) equipped with processing power and the ability to communicate can either wholly or partially be used to solve the problem. It was this question that excited Wan and was the endpoint of a journey he had started more than a decade earlier.

Dr. Wan had taken a circuitous path on his way to entering the health care system and his current research focus. After graduation from Wuhan University in China, he moved to the United States to continue his studies in information sciences. He eventually landed a position at the University of California at Berkeley, where he began his work in the world of sensor-based research. His early focus was in the automobile industry, which at the time was experiencing its own revolution in information sciences through the growth of inboard computers.

Wan had an unusual vision, focused on a world of connected information resources, controlled through a diverse collection of microcontrollers, linked through wired/wireless communications, and ultimately managed by decision-support programs. His first health care product was the Magic Medicine Cabinet (MMC), which, when introduced in 1999, represented a clever preview of where the health industry could head. The MMC was in reality a convergence of new thinking from the computer industry in the areas of radio frequency tagging, face/speech recognition, and closed-loop information processing. It also represented an intermarriage of the virtual with the physical. As described by Wan, the MMC would, "enable consumers to:

- Perform routine physical care, such as reminding and ensuring one to take the right medication and tracking vital signs;
- Access up-to-date personalized health information; and
- Interact online with physicians, pharmacists, and other professional care providers."[1]

Wan believed the connection of individuals to an environment was critical, with health care being a place where the virtual and physical could operate in tandem. When a person stepped up to the

MMC, it would perform a scan to determine who they were (through facial recognition) and then provide feedback to the individual on a screen embedded in the front of the medicine cabinet. The MMC would then begin interactions based on the actions of the individual and guide the individual through the compliance process—ensuring they followed the directions relevant to their problem by reminding them to take their medications or even stopping them if they began to take the wrong one.

An Automated Feedback Loop

On one hand, the MMC was dealing with the issue of facility. While the historic center for health encounters has been the physician's office, the hospital, and other health treatment facilities, the MMC questioned whether a physical portal could be built to effectively move the location of the health care encounter to any place or any time.

It also addressed the issue of information consolidation and processing. The MMC could communicate with a number of external sensors, with a human user and the outside world—and it could act on that information based on certain rules of the road that it understood. If the MMC felt that you were about to do something wrong it told you so and recommended you reconsider your action. The MMC had become your intelligent assistant and overseer. Yet the idea that devices could have intelligence built into them was not something Wan invented, nor was it an innovation of the health care industry. Because along with the growth of the microprocessor another giant appeared on the scene in the 1970s—*microcontrollers*—and the computer had become transparent and showing up in a number of different places and industries. Information was being managed around us and without our help. Andy Peter and his colleagues in the auto repair industry already understood that world, and you live with it every time you drive your car. And it starts with an incredibly small piece of silicon with an unusual amount of power.

The microcontroller is basically a miniature and limited computer wrapped in a small package. Whereas a personal computer requires a number of supporting mechanisms (such as a keyboard and a monitor), a microcontroller is comfortable working in isolation. It operates according to a set of predefined ways, reacting to its environment in limited, preprogrammed ways.

And although you are probably not even aware of it—the microcontroller has become one of your biggest friends. If you have a clothes dryer or refrigerator in your house, chances are there is a microcontroller inside of it happily overseeing the appliance to make sure it is doing what it is supposed to do.

As an information appliance, the MMC was closer to the model typically used within microcontroller environments, although with a noticeable benefit: flexibility. The MMC shared the characteristic of these other environments (e.g., the control unit housed within your car) in that it can react to signals within its "system." It also had the ability to dynamically adjust to new information resources and be reprogrammed on the fly.

But there was more. Your car and its embedded computer technologies generally react to almost everyone the same way. Whether you, your friend or spouse drives your car its internal systems think and act the same way. The MMC is different—it focused on the unique needs of the individual. When the MMC recognized an individual, it progressed beyond the simplistic one-size-fits-all model, building its reactions based on the individual's unique profile using a combination of clever decision-support applications. It would, for example, remind you that you had already taken your medication had you done something as innocuous as just picking up the bottle.

This idea of linking the reactions of a system (the MMC) to the individual's actions balanced by what the system believes is normal and appropriate behavior is the textbook definition of decision support. If the patient takes the wrong medication, the MMC understands the error and reacts. The MMC is therefore providing the patient with a level of automated decision support, guiding what it understands to be appropriate actions—and flagging those it believes are in error.

With any closed-loop approach, the key is in how the control parameters are defined. The solution to this problem would be found through another major innovation of our movement to PHC—the emerging field of sensor-based decision making, with some of earliest examples of this way of thinking dating back to the 1950s.

Moving Inside the Body

The pacemaker is a device with a rich history. Research into the causes and treatments of cardiac disease has been robust and long-standing—the illness is one of the most critical and expensive health issues confronting our society—with the invention and evolution of the pacemaker being one of its great achievements.

Ultimately the pacemaker is a powerful example of how to attack the problems of the body through a man-made technology. It reacts and performs its actions as part of the system of the heart and it does so without your guidance on what it should be doing or how it should do it. It has become an autonomic engine. But it did not start that way.

The modern pacemaker has grown from a complex and bulky connection of wires and sensors to an elegant example of packaged information technology. The story of its recent and rapid evolution began with the interest and talents of a young engineer from Minnesota named Earl Bakken.

Born in Minneapolis in 1924, Bakken graduated with a degree in electrical engineering from the University of Minnesota. Through one of life's many chance encounters and his wife (a hospital worker), he became aware of the decision-making questions of the health care industry and was about to focus his formidable creative skills on "engineering" problems in medicine. Along the way he connected with Dr. C. Walton Lillehei and an industry was about to be revolutionized. The seed for the Medtronic Corporation was just planted.

The opportunity Lillehei presented Bakken was huge for such a young, albeit enterprising, engineer. In 1957, pacemakers were well-established medical devices used in the intensive care units of the nation's larger hospitals. A state-of-the-art pacemaker involved an awkward combination of technologies that required a source of AC power to run, was limited in application, and was clearly not portable (at least not by today's standards).

This was a test for Bakken and would require some creative redesigning. In his autobiography, Bakken described the event.

> Back at the garage, I dug out a back issue of *Popular Electronics* magazine in which I recalled seeing a circuit for an electronic, transistorized metronome. The circuit transmitted clicks through a loudspeaker; the rate of the clicks could be adjusted to fit the music. I simply modified that circuit and placed it, without the loudspeaker, in a four-inch-square, inch-and-thick metal box with terminals and switches on the outside—and that, as they say, was that.[2]

But few people, including Lillehei, anticipated what would happen next.

Within a few weeks of initial discussions between Bakken and Lillehei, the first "portable" pacemaker was created and taped to a patient's chest.

As you would expect, Bakken and his colleagues were not the only group interested in how to extend the power of this device. And they were still left with a couple of big questions to answer, with one of the most pressing being how to supply power. Electrical current coming through a wall plate has several limitations, especially when you consider the device is attached to a person and the person may want or need to move around. The Bakken solution was simple—use a 9V battery.

But Drs. William Chardack and Andrew Gage, at the Veterans Administration in Buffalo, New York, had another idea. Why not use a different type of energy cell from the standard rechargeable technologies of the day as the power source and take the pacemaker off the chest wall of the patient?

Chardack and his colleagues designed the implantable pacemaker and along the way created one of the great innovations of machine-based intelligence—we were moving from outside to inside. For the first time in history, the medical community had the ability to augment the functions of the body through a man-made internal device. Pandora's box was open and the pacemaker, along with a number of other coming revolutions in the computer industry, would help redefine the roles of sensors in health care and show us how to enter the complex mechanical systems housed within us. The pacemaker had demonstrated that it was possible to build intelligence that could be added inside of the human—and how that intelligence could work in concert with one of its most complex systems.

The speed of the story began to accelerate through an increasing convergence of ideas, technology solutions, and applications. Along the way, the modern Medtronic has slowly evolved into a next generation computer/information technology firm. Where it was once a developer of devices that were used to keep the heart beating, Medtronic is now a manager of information—helping the body through a complex integration of technical components (including microprocessors and communications) and applications. The Internet, also dating back to 1957, would converge with Medtronic by the end of the twentieth century and define yet another enabler to machine-based solutions. Pacemakers could now talk through communication lines back to other systems and an almost unlimited number of other applications. Where will we be going next?

The question of how far to go introduces one of the final aspects of machine-based intelligence, the growth of artificial intelligence (AI). And like almost all the converging forces of nature behind the PHC revolution, AI began quietly and without much public attention.

Setting the Stage

As one of the original code breakers in the famous Bletchley Park, Alan Turing was accustomed to working with abstract problems. Among his many accomplishments, Turing is known for his theoretical design of the computer as a mathematical machine—the relationship of functions that helped define our modern computer architecture.

Turing also provided society with a number of seminal ideas on machine intelligence. One of the more interesting conceptual issues was related to AI. As described[3] in his 1950 article, "Computing Machinery and Intelligence," Turing proposed a relatively simple dilemma to test the ability of a questioner to decide whether the answers to his or her queries came from a person or a machine. If the questioner could not decipher whether the answers came from a computer, then the computer had successfully demonstrated "artificial intelligence."

Although a basic construct, it raises issues across a number of domains—many of which we will wrestle with for generations to come. The general ideas are based on the notion that a computer, with its abilities to manage an almost unlimited number of interconnections, could perform logical analysis in the same way or sometimes better than a person. In the case of the Magic Medicine Cabinet, the ability of the computer to recognize the person is a current example of this line of research—we do it instinctively (recognize our friends and neighbors, for example). Could we build that same capability into a computer application? The MMC demonstrated that yes, we could, at least in the small micro-world of pharmaceuticals.

In general, the evolution of AI in medicine has been exciting to watch, with a short history of interesting characters and achievement—and represents the greatest long-term potential for change in the field. But the community of AI researchers face a number of formidable obstacles, with the question of how to automatically classify information being near the top of the list.

And it starts with a basic challenge for our machine partners—our human/animal ability to understand and put context in our environment.

Our brains allow us to do things and deal with information in ways that are sometimes hard to describe. Think for a moment about the process of reading this book and how you parse through words and build meaning. Or think of how effortlessly you comprehend the words of someone that you know. You would be surprised at the amount of "understanding" you have that incorporates a mixture of sight and sounds—or is based on your ability to think ahead and match patterns. Now imagine how difficult this problem is for machines that do not have the benefit of the language imprinting we received as small children.

Luckily for us, the challenge of "reading" the signals of your heart was ultimately a bit easier than understanding the nuances of human language.

Automatic Classification

Almost everyone who has ever visited a doctor's office has heard of the electrocardiogram (EKG) machine. With the modern version having roots dating back to the early twentieth century, the EKG provided an elegant way of measuring the electrical signals in your body and highlighting the health (or weaknesses) of your heart.

By the 1960s, the EKG became a staple of the medical practice as a new class of physicians with the skills to translate the subtle movements of lines across the paper to "read" the condition of the patient's heart emerged. Irregular signals tended to characterize problems, with these signals ranging from difficult to easy-to-characterize, at least for the trained eye. Eventually, the ability to read the output of the EKG became an accepted part of the medical practice and was one of the many "skills" a health professional possessed.

Something funny happened to the EKG in the 1990s. Suddenly, the machine began providing its own analysis of the signals—effectively giving the interpretation of what it was reading within the patient without requiring the intervention of a physician or a trained technologist. The EKG had become "smart" and had begun incorporating a decision-support program analogous to the machine-intelligence claims that had begun with Turing and continued through the decades with varying levels of success.

The era of technology-based decision support had begun. While no one was watching, the packaging of a closed-loop model within the EKG represented a real-world solution to a problem that appeared as one of the holy grails of the industry. But it still begs the question: could we make computers think?

Computer-Based Decision Making

The premise is a simple one. Medical professionals are required to comprehend and recall a tremendous amount of information. The complexity of our bodies, the ways conditions tend to be masked by other conditions—layering in ways that make the process of deciding what is what—seem more like an art or inherent skill than a science. This complexity, which on its surface appears to fit within the confines of some type of if-then model, became the subject of a variety of research programs dating back to the birth of the artificial intelligence community. One of the most ambitious undertakings was the work on the Internist project by Drs. Jack Meyers and Harry Pople.

The Internist was chartered to attack the "big" problem of medicine—defining a solution from the often confusing array of signs and symptoms to establish a differential diagnosis. The problem seemed straightforward enough.

A disease usually presents a typical set of symptoms and values. Coupling the physician's observations and information gleaned from the data side of medicine—lab values, pathology studies, radiology results, and the like—a more complete diagnosis can be made.

But there is a problem: diseases can cluster around one another, resulting in a confusing picture of what is right and wrong. Remember the discussion on establishing relevant data points? If it sounds familiar to the problem being addressed by the Meyers and Pople team—or how to construct a solution based on seemingly unconnected observations or data points—it does for good reason. It is exactly the same type of problem we are facing in the post-genomic world of almost infinite data. So what is the solution that they created?

The founding team of Meyers and Pople was, on the surface, an odd couple. Their partnership was one based on the symbiotic value of the expert (Meyers) and the developer (Pople) merging their knowledge of medicine with new thinking on how to program a computer. At the time, the idea that the domain knowledge of a professional—the data, heuristics, and problem-solving process—would be valuable to an application developer was untested. Knowledge-based medicine was a theory but definitely not something that was viewed as being relevant to the everyday medical practice.

Nonetheless the results of their collaboration were impressive. Although not designed to solve the most fundamental problems (the general view of the team was that if a physician was unable to diagnosis the basic issues, then they should not be in the profession), the Internist did appear to handle the most complex interactions in a way that at least rivaled the best of the specialists. This positioned the Internist as a natural adjunct to the primary care practice of medicine, allowing the frontline players to diagnose with the sophistication of an expert. While the concept seemed like a winner, a couple of problems prevented the Internist from hitting the mainstream. One was the state of computing.

Given its connection to a machine (it ran on a computer), the Internist required a certain level of sophistication on the part of its target users—physicians with a reasonable base of medical training and experience in computers. Unfortunately this sophistication was in short supply when Meyers and Pople brought their seminal research to the broader community of medicine. Although computers are today an everyday part of our lives, they were generally unknown for the vast majority of people when Meyers and Pople began their journey in the 1970s.

Ultimately what Meyers and Pople unleashed was similar to the Defense Advanced Research Projects Agency (DARPA) and the Sputnik—and the drive in science and engineering to create, among other great end products, the eventual Internet. Meyers and Pople were leading the evolution of a different type of computer application—one based on the knowledge and data confronting professionals doing their jobs—and they helped push the embryonic artificial intelligence community ahead. We were, thanks to their unheralded efforts, beginning to attack a new conceptual problem. Computers could be great adding machines, as IBM and others demonstrated in the 1960s, but they could clearly do more—and Meyers and Pople were showing us how this new form of computer application could impact something as critical as medical diagnostics.

For a number of people, the idea that a computer would be used to provide the sole diagnosis of a problem is a future they would prefer to avoid. Having the comfort of the human-to-human contact—being able to sit with their physician in their office and listening to their voice—is not only important, it provided a sense of confidence that the correct answer was being provided to them. They wanted comfort and truth and the only way it could be realized was through the personal interactions with their physician.

But in our world of complex data, and with the knowledge we are gaining on the infinite variability of our gene/environment interactions, we will have no choice but to accept and embrace this increasing focus on machine-based thinking. As I discussed earlier, we will need to have a variety of knowledge utilities to survive, as the era of PHC will demand. And guess what—it is already happening around you. The future of human/machine solutions has arrived in almost every application of industry.

Next time you make a phone call or get online, try imagining which technologies are being used to support your voice or data connection. Also, next time you get a blood test, consider the automated technologies and analysis being used to read your sample.

Lucky for almost all of us, we do not need to understand even the basic theories behind these inventions. Computers and computer technology operate as our partners, ensuring these now ubiquitous forms of technology work and work well.

The conclusions are basic. Decision-support solutions are getting stronger every day as part of the silent evolution of the information marketplace—and the growth of the knowledge economy. They make our technical solutions work for us in the background, often correcting problems before we realize they even exist.

So where will we be heading beyond these computer-based decision-support systems? For a hint of what the future may look like, ask anyone younger than thirty what he thinks of DOOM from id Software.

Get ready for a new reality.

Entering a Virtual World

One of the most fascinating developments in the computer-game industry has been the growth and use of immersive computer environments. The idea is a simple one.

You peer into the computer screen and through the interaction of keys, joysticks, and other input devices are suddenly thrust inside the middle of an artificial world—a world totally constructed on the new media of the computer. Existing only as a digital creation, the virtual world invites you to join the action of the game far beyond the board games of the past.

To those of us who grew up with computers in the 1970s and 1980s, our concept of media tended to come in different shades of green, with a black background providing the canvas. This reality changed dramatically during the 1990s as graphics and graphical engines invaded the personal computer space and rise of sophisticated gaming machines (Xbox, PlayStation, etc.). Where heavy graphics were once the stuff of legends (and incredibly expensive computer environments), it suddenly, and almost overnight, was everywhere and on every desktop.

As with most new ideas involving teenagers, the movement was criticized and misunderstood by adults and, notwithstanding their concerns, became widely successful. Artificial gaming worlds became the equivalent of the hot rods of the 1950s with a new vocabulary and packs of enthusiastic supporters. The names of the early games are now legendary with DOOM being one of the earliest and Halo the most recent "hit."

As their popularity rose, the negative consequences linked to these new game environments became the fodder of urban legends. Rumor mills discussed, although never proved, a connection between violence, aggression, and practically every ailment related to the common teen experience. Many people criticized this new generation of entertainment as a dummying down of society. While the old board games like Monopoly forced us to use our minds and creative energies, the new generation of computer games, the argument went, transformed our children in something akin to a drug-induced haze. Instead of creating miniature Einsteins, we were producing megazombies.

Luckily, not everyone shared this view.

A number of our more creative colleagues saw the possibilities that emanated from the teenager's gaming environments. Why not use these artificial worlds to support the training requirements of industry, with medicine and the airline communities in the lead? To these industry groups, the potential of artificial worlds and all-encompassing media foreshadowed newer learning environments, something they desperately needed but could rarely afford to acquire.

Consider the alternatives: training doctors about new procedures with real patients is a dangerous proposition, just as using real planes to teach a pilot the nuances of flying is prohibitively expensive.

How confident would you feel knowing the surgeon scheduled to operate on you tomorrow will be performing her first-ever procedure on a live patient? And just how confident would you feel if, on your trip, your airline decided to seat you in some experimental plane for your cross-country flight from Boston to Los Angeles? If these scenarios were real, more than likely you would cancel both the surgery and your flight.

In the end, the immersive environment represents an example of another convergence and ultimately personalization—this time within the computer industry and a collection of creative designers who attack real problems in education and training. Lucky for us flying in planes or having surgery, the group proved to be tremendously successful and their work is now part of standard training programs of many emerging areas. But this future is just starting to unfold, with the pursuit of education being only the first of what will be many applications.

One of these more interesting future uses of the human map is its ability to be used within therapeutic environments, as I highlighted with the brain map. Through the integration of data on us (acquired through our various data-harvesting technologies) with new ways of delivering therapies, the health care community will have the tools to provide us with individualized solutions—not simply the ones driven by the one-size-fits-all models. The net is that the immersive reality concepts of the game world will be entering health care through a completely different way of thinking about personalization. DOOM enters the operating room.

Consider the issues of a surgeon. Surgery is often a complicated affair for everyone involved—including the surgeon, the supporting professional staff, the hospital, and the patient. But the world of our surgical professionals is about to change. With the introduction of virtual environments and robotic controls, it really is time to enter the world of science fiction. But guess what—this is already happening at your local hospital.

A Convergence of Ideas

Had you been experiencing hip pain in the mid-1990s, you may have bumped into Russell Taylor, who, at the time, worked at IBM's Watson research labs. His interests were unusual for a computer company—he focused on how to optimize the fit of an artificial hip within a patient. His solutions were also clever—a robot that would assist a surgeon with the complex procedure of drilling into the bone to replace it with an artificial joint. He, along with several colleagues, believed that they could help the surgeon do a better job.

But Taylor was not a physician. He was a member of the engineering community and a world expert in robotics technologies. What did he know about medicine?

As described throughout this book, our bodies are balanced and complex machines. We have a standard set of linkages allowing it to work well in concert—with the connection of bones in our joints being one of the most important. When you suffer from certain forms of arthritis or have been injured severely, the integrity of the mechanical connection of one bone to another may be compromised, leading to a loss of function and persistent pain. Enter Robodoc from Taylor and his colleagues as the new and better mousetrap for orthopedic surgery.

The innovation of Taylor and his colleagues merged a number of converging threads I discussed throughout my multichapter discussion on technology. First, he had to amass data on the patient, obtained through a number of the data acquisition programs. Taylor then had to utilize that data to create a useful representation of a 3-D world—the underlying microcommunity of the body and a human map.

Next, he constructed a virtual reality model of the now 3-D structure and connected it to a set of sensors. The sensors would, in turn, help drive the actions of a device that would guide the surgeon along in a procedure.

Taylor had, in attacking a problem facing the orthopedic surgeon (and hip replacement procedures), integrated almost every technical element of the emerging systems of PHC within the construct of a simple (although difficult-to-perform) operation. The patient suffered from a bad hip so the surgeon would remove the damaged parts and replace it with a titanium implant.

In the end what Taylor and the team accomplished was valuable for the patient and represented an incredible feat of innovation spanning data mining through sensors. As my discourse on data harvesting discussed, the questions of data collection are by no means answered. The volume and magnitude of data in health care are increasing in size and expanse on an almost daily basis. Lacking the ability to navigate within a digital data world would have ended the discussion—the 3-D structures of the body needed an appropriate way of being described, and the computer and its ability to model were the only way to do it. Paper and other forms of storage were complete nonstarters for solving the problem facing Taylor.

Next was the real-time integration of sensor data. As you noticed in the discussion on the pacemaker, we have achieved amazing feats in manufacturing technologies, with the ability to create smaller and smaller form factors that operate flawlessly and as part of a larger system.

But Taylor's problems did not end with the technology—he also needed to have his sensor guide the surgical process, letting the surgeon know when the cut was made at the appropriate levels to optimize the physical connection of the artificial joint with the patient's remaining bone. This linkage of information and sensor data during an operating-room procedure was risky and rewarding—and it also broke new ground.

Last, putting it all together was probably the single biggest hurdle, especially considering the issues of how one can change the sociological world of the operating room and break the habits of the surgeon and medical team. It is a problem that is being addressed through the fundamental rethinking of the health care system.

As the work of Taylor and a number of the other research scientists I have mentioned earlier highlight, the systems, people, and applications of PHC are already starting to appear around us. And they are leading to a transformational event that author Malcolm Gladwell understands.

He should—he educated a number of us on the topic a few years back.

Notes

1. Dadong Wan, "Personalized ubiquitous commerce: An application perspective," *Kluwer Academic Publishers*, 2004.

2. Earl E. Bakken, "One man's full life," Medtronic, 1999.

3. Originally published by Oxford University Press on behalf of *MIND* (the journal of the Mind Association), 59, no. 236, (1950): 433–60.

PART IV

A LIFE REBORN

Medicine is a calling, not a business.

—SIR WILLIAM OSLER

I n 2000, one of the best sellers in the business community was written by Malcolm Gladwell. It was called *The Tipping Point: How Little Things Can Make a Big Difference.*

The chapters of his book emphasized that nearly all transformations experienced a cycle of growth that eventually led to a "tipping point" where it was no longer possible to return to the old way of doing things. Call it achieving critical mass, an inflection, or the tipping point, and the impact is the same—the world would now be a different place.

Gladwell's book became required reading for anyone interested in how and why things changed and should be a wakeup call for the health care industry. Whether the various institutions that populate the medical community like it or not, seismic shifts do occur. Sometimes the winds of change blow softly, barely recognizable, but at some point, the seemingly covert brewing transforms into a "tipping point," creating a new reality.

I would argue that society is at the beginning of this phase for health care with the converging forces I have described poised to redefine the industry. And as the eICU, CTSNet, and the pacemaker are demonstrating, it is probably already starting to occur.

How will this tipping point impact the health care of patients and the various professionals and institutions that provide services in the systems of personalize health care (PHC)? The changes will include a few casualties along the way—along with a wealth of new opportunities for enterprising individuals.

From the demise of such great brands and companies as the Digital Electric Corporation (DEC) and the slow decline of the Ford Motor Company, we should have grown accustomed to the fact that wholesale changes in industry dynamics and leadership are the norm. As history has so well documented, most groups do not survive such overwhelming transitions.

Anyone who doubts that reality should try to find an old Kodak film canister in a drawer. It's doubtful you'll find one.

Death of a Giant

Incorporated at the end of the nineteenth century, the Kodak Corporation had been a historic market and thought leader of the photography industry. Its founder, George Eastman, turned the camera and pictures into a common ritual of society.

His motto was simple: "You press the button, we do the rest."

By the middle of the twentieth century, Kodak had become an example of how innovative thinking could build success, which translated to literally tens of thousands of new jobs and a vibrant economy for Rochester, New York. Sadly for the many employees of Kodak, however, that same set of converging forces as described in parts II and III were set to define their own tipping point for the world of photography, and by the end of the twentieth century, they did so with dramatic consequences.

Whereas even ten years ago the standard for taking pictures was film, today digital cameras and digital pictures have become commonplace, with cameras now built into everything from cell phones to personal digital assistants (PDAs).

Digital picture taking also represents another example of the forces of personalization—you take the picture, you process it, and you mail it around without needing a darkroom. While this is great news for consumers, it was bad for Kodak and other companies that manufacture camera film. Digital technologies tend to operate in the world of charges and particles—not the paper and chemistry of the old Kodak.

A parallel transformation has also occurred in the music industry, where the former analog versions of the LP and cassette tapes have basically bowed to their digital replacements, the music CD and the emerging virtual world of MP3. Music, just like pictures and now even video, has evolved into a new form of digital currency. Digital change is happening everywhere.

Who will be impacted by the convergence of the digital world and health care?

As our discussion on the emergence of virtual communities highlighted, the framework of community is in a process of reinvention, with the old notions of proximity having less and less relevance as more people worldwide hop on the Internet. This change is leading people to redefine their communities more by collections of people with common interests—and less by their neighborhood.

The experiences of the eICU and CTSNet have demonstrated the impact that information technology and the Internet can have on the meaning and interactions of a community of users in health care. Where else will it evolve?

I will need to start this discussion with a few definitions. Get ready for a new hospital.

Redefinitions

The historic symbols of the health care industry have been the hospital and the physician. The hospital has emerged as the single most visible identifier of the market. Its presence often towers over small towns, appearing on the horizon as the modern equivalent of church steeples centuries back. It is also fast becoming the largest single employer in our rural economies.

The other symbol of our industry is the white-coated physician who manages the "process" of delivering treatments to patients.

Physicians have obtained an aura and almost mythical status as the associated "priest" to the churchlike presence of the hospital.

These symbols of our industry have evolved during a period where not much was known about disease or even how to treat it. The movement initiated by the publication of Osler's *Principles and Practice of Medicine* was a great start in migrating to a scientific foundation with substance, but it came into play far after these other institutions had defined their positions of power in the community. And also, yes, these symbols have become substantial in size and influence, and like all large organizations, will resist change.

As you might expect given the increasing power of our knowledge economy, both of these groups will experience major transformations as society moves toward a system of PHC. The preceding chapters provided you with an introduction to the vast number of scientific and technical innovations. How have these innovations impacted our current systems of health care delivery?

The answer is that they are starting, but they are dealing with a number of legacy issues. The hospitals of yesterday were designed for a period in time where diseases were viewed as an outbreak—and not as the result of a complex interaction of variables occurring over time and in concert with the genetic makeup of an individual. Disease in our earlier history was a near spiritual mystery of the body.

Although many mysteries remain, medicine is at least at the point where we not only appreciate but understand that a certain cause-and-effect relationship exists in how disease impacts our bodies and are moving beyond the ideas that framed the basis of hospital design in the nineteenth century. As I highlighted earlier, disease and health can now be discussed around their fundamental mechanical and mission-oriented drivers.

Given the evolving paradigm for health, is the current architecture of the hospital the best way of managing disease and health—and does it represent what we would create today as we embark on a restructuring of the health care industry?

The answer is simple: no.

Relearning Health

Before I begin discussing the new facility architecture, I need to reorient our mapping of a system that that I call the *health/life* model. The components of this model demonstrate how our health status is actually the result of a number of ways of living—and that we need to begin understanding how each of these "slices" of the pie may and probably should come with their own collections of tested and accurate sources of knowledge and supporting professionals. Remember my earlier discussion on truth and confidence? Get ready for a number of misleading claims and a need to figure out who really does *know* what is good for you—and even has the depth of knowledge to give you advice.

So, as you might expect, the fully evolved systems of PHC will require more than a doctor of medicine to support its delivery. Health will become a combination of system management models ranging from basic issues of mechanics to the way you interact with your neighbors. And luckily for us we at least have a starting point for the model—the body as a *machine*.

This first piece of the health/life model interconnects our bodies as a mechanical device to the challenges of managing health and disease. I like to call it our "system maintenance" function given its obvious correlation back to supporting the body's many systems. Remember the discussion concerning the tragic accident of Christopher Reeve? His cascading system errors were the ultimate testimony to the importance of the connected systems of our bodies—and how critical it is that we have both knowledge and skilled professions working with us.

Who are the professionals driving this system-maintenance practice? They are the physicians through nurses and an emerging array of allied and alternative health professionals that provide treatments to us today. They are also most often engaged after a condition has been noticed or a trauma occurs through elaborate and generally sound ways of ensuring that we receive the most current thinking on how to keep the machines of our bodies alive.

The next section of the health/life model is "physical tuning." Physical tuning refers to the organized use of physical activity to strengthen and enhance the body's natural defenses. When was the last time you received a prescription for monitored exercise as part of your treatment program from your physician? Maybe you did, but more than likely you did not and should have.

One of the end products of the increasing automation and technical growth of our society is immobility. People simply do not walk around much anymore and are engaged in far less exercise and physical activity than we were a century earlier. Our ingenuity in discovering more efficient ways of transporting ourselves or doing things with the help of physical extenders, such as cars, power saws, and even the fairly new Segway device, are but a few of the culprits.

The bad news is that the literally millions of years of evolution supporting our bodies was not designed with this thinking in mind—they were built to manage the energy consumption and storage of energy in our bodies when we walked around in a hostile environment. Going to the shopping center to pick out the food for your next meal is far easier than having to constantly scour the woods for things that are edible and nutritious—and a lot less stressful that fighting with a variety of dangerous animals that were looking at you as part of their next meal.

The next component of the health/life model is the function of "energy renewal," and is something we actively manage on a daily basis, although not necessarily well. On one level, it can be interpreted as basic nutrition—providing the body with a proper mix of nutrients required by your cells to survive and prosper.

How well would our cars run if we insisted on filling the gas tank with water? The answer is that they would immediately stop. Our bodies are a far more tolerant machine than a car engine, for example, accepting abuse that other machines would find fatal. Following an unhealthy diet and then maintaining it in its unhealthy state for many years may not kill you immediately. But you can be sure that it will alter the mission-driven potential of your body and reduce your future productive years.

On a completely different level, "energy renewal" is defined as the process of rebuilding that sleep and general resting provides. Our brains are a complicated engine of control, overflowing with massive amounts of data it must manage. Our muscles also require their own period of rebuild, as any body builder can explain in detail. The need to recharge and sleep is a necessary part of the cycle.

The final management function of the health/life model is "social support," and is the most abstract to define despite impacting almost all areas of our lives. Through the growth of communities, to blending within the relationships of our families and friends, we exist within a mosaic of complex social environments. The relationships we form with our friends, family, religions, co-workers, teammates, and so on, are critical elements in how we react to and manage disease and grow our health. While we typically define environmental variables through obvious encounters like second-hand smoke, or Love Canal and Chernobyl, we often overlook another of the more critical components— how we relate to and are supported by others.

In summary, it is the combination of these activities—systems maintenance, physical tuning, energy renewal, and social support—that comprise the puzzle pieces of the new delivery systems of PHC. As you delve into the lower-level requirements of these unique areas, you begin to understand the requirement for a variety of professionals to support your health evolution. The physician, while important, will not be alone anymore. And yes, nutritionists will become incredibly valuable to you—or at least should—along with your personal trainer.

How will each of these professionals accomplish their unique health missions? The answer is through information, tons of it, and the constant checking of your personal data values against your own set of personal averages.

In the chapters to follow I explore various ways our health care system should evolve. It is a future with deep roots in the past, connected to a variety of other industry transformations. You should probably get ready for a few new faces to gain prominence in our lives, as well. Remember, Microsoft was not a division of IBM, and Toyota was not born in Detroit. And where did Google come from anyway?

CHAPTER 10

THE INFORMATION HIGHWAY

O N APRIL 27, 2004, President George W. Bush signed an executive order creating the position of National Health Information Technology Coordinator. This new post, chaired by Dr. David Brailer, was created as a first step in constructing a national system for assembling comprehensive patient information to allow accurate, quick, and easy transmission of information among health providers. Creating a national "highway" infrastructure for health care information is a major undertaking intended to benefit society in a manner analogous to how the national highway system is built for transportation.

Turn the clock back fifty years and you will notice a number of interesting parallels.

On June 29, 1956, President Dwight Eisenhower signed the national Interstate and Defense Highways Act, which began the largest public works project in the history of the United States. The results of the act included a roughly $25 billion investment on more than 40,000 miles of interstate highways covering the length and breadth of the continental United States. It was the culmination of the grand period of the automobile and an official recognition that the transportation industry, which in the previous century had been dominated by the railroad, was now under the control of a very different machine, offering an even greater set of opportunities—the car.

The motor vehicle had officially become the first choice for "personal" movement, and the second half of the twentieth century began with the clatter of earthmovers and dump trucks.

Without the guidance and support of the federal government, the design and implementation of a highway network would more than likely have resulted in the chaos of connecting small roads optimized around what each city and state required. Without federal leadership, the highway system might have succeeded in linking Philadelphia to Pittsburgh or Los Angeles to San Francisco, but would have been a mess for travelers trying to drive from Philadelphia to Los Angeles, for example. Humans, as we can all appreciate from a basic knowledge of history, tend to cluster in local communities and will do what is best for themselves first and then maybe their neighbors next. Thinking big has never been our strong point, which a "national" network of highways that optimized the entire U.S. transportation network would require.

So the geometric rise of the automobile, combined with the growth of an uncontrolled highway system, forced the hand of the federal government—and the eventual move by President Eisenhower in 1956 to bring order to the chaos. Someone needed to define the national highway infrastructure and who better than the federal government, with the Interstate and Defense Highways Act, born nearly half a century ago, leading the charge.

For advocates of state's rights it may have sounded like yet another move to big government. In an analogous way, society is at the initial stages of watching the government grapple with defining standard for our proposed National Health Information Network (NHIN). Similar to how our early road systems developed, the project has already begun at the state and local level through the emergence of the Regional Health Information Organizations (RHIO) and the growth of smaller community-based health networks.

But it is also clear that, just as with the national highway system for moving vehicles, a uniform set of standards will be necessary to construct the NHIN and make it work across the country and for everyone. But despite the fact that the overall goals might be similar, improving the mobility of cars and creating lanes of communication, the construction of the NHIN will not necessarily follow the same rules as those used for building streets and expressways.

First, the NHIN will not have to be funded by the federal government.

Most of our health care system operates through a loose collection of providers, paid for by a mixture of consumers, business, and government. Given the increasing complexity and types of information resources, the movement/compliance to a certain standard is something the government alone cannot force upon the systems of health care.

Second, the communication system will not be hardwired. Certainly, for any industry standard it is critical that the right handshakes occur between parts that fit together. Lacking standards, for example, we would be unable to access our bank accounts via an automatic teller machine (ATM) in machines not owned by our bank. Imagine the confusion if these transfers were not done correctly—your cash could wind up in someone else's account.

The potential for improving the quality of care we receive is one of the many important reasons to have a series of connected information resources. It also ensures our health records are not lost despite all the moves we make in our lives. Imagine the nightmare of being involved in an accident, arriving unconscious to a hospital emergency department with a prior history of allergic reactions to some of the most common antibiotics. With a little luck, you may live through the incident, but you can rest assured your medical care would have been improved had your attending physicians had access to your prior health records.

So yes, standards will have to be defined to ensure the right connections are made—but they will have to be created with the recognition that the ways the connections will occur will sometimes vary.

Have you ever found yourself in a place where absolutely no one understood your language? In that situation even getting the simplest idea communicated from one person to another can be extremely difficult.

Defining a Standard

I am reasonably confident that you do not know anyone who can speak to you in the Jurchen language. Jurchen is one of the world's extinct languages, once spoken by a community of people living on the plains of central China.

To be fair to those former speakers of this elegant dialect, the creation of unique languages is a wonderful example of creative thinking by evolving human as we migrated and settled the world. It is much easier to transfer ideas from one person to another when both individuals speak the same language, which clearly aided in the social organization of our emerging and evolving society. But what happens when this reality of our social organization (i.e., our tendencies to form local tribes and communities within regions) expands across vast continents and creates isolated populations and, eventually, different languages?

The answer is you have a mess on your hands, and especially in a globally connected world. Whose label for "water" is the correct one to use? Is it *acqua* as an Italian would say or 근해 in Korean?

Society is faced with a similar question of compatibility in our movement to a system of electronic record keeping for health care, albeit one that luckily does not have the emotional baggage the language debate often carries. Our problem of compatibility in health care, while still immense, will come down to the issues of electronic representation and inclusion.

Another major obstacle: the sources of this data may actually emanate from literally thousands of sources, with the potential to add literally millions of variables to the final equation and health-data repository.

Your Personal Health Record

So where does this journey start? The first step, at least one that impacts the most people, will be through the growth of a personal health record. This personal health record will become the single most important component of the systems of PHC and the way the various members of our emerging health team will communicate with us, themselves, and over time.

With that in mind, let's return to the beauty of Google and the general concepts of Web searching. Search engines like Google have found that the best solutions for answering our information questions are dynamic and must support the reality that the sources of data are constantly changing.

When you place a search query on the Internet, the search engine parses through the Internet's rich information objects to locate the best possible matches, ranking its findings as it presents them to you on your computer's monitor. Consider how this thinking could impact the value of electronic patient records, as well as data repositories, as a source of all available medical information.

If the NHIN eventually builds upon the same models of connected information nodes as the Internet, and the various data repositories of the health care industry become connected to this health infrastructure, then it is quite probable the connection of a patient's record with a repository of scientific information will operate in a manner similar to how the search engine community works with today's Internet. The future patient record will represent a dynamic collection of information resources assembled on the fly and featuring a wealth of information sources.

On one level, it is clear the medical community will need to combine, for instance, all the treatment data and information we have on the various and evolving mission-related elements of people's life. The medical community is beginning to appreciate, for example, that certain clusters of genetics in an individual may result in specific downstream events. This element of prediction could therefore be an accepted part of what is contained in your record, with an ability to do a little forward thinking on how your health may change over time, or how a disease may progress through its own evolutionary stages.

But along with these "traditional" forms of health data, we will also have the opportunity to include broader collections of data points, even those whose relationship to our current health status we do not understand. Remember the story of Love Canal?

Before we examine this issue further, it is time to return to the transistor and another powerful example of an event and set of downstream consequences.

Power of Prediction

In 1947, William Shockley and his colleagues at Bell Laboratories made a discovery that would have an impact far beyond the imaginations of most people who had reviewed their eventual patent and the description of this innovative creation, the transistor. On one level, the Shockley invention appeared primitive. It created a simple electronic gate. Push the current one way, it opened. Push the current other way, it closed. Interesting, yes, but it was not some type of life-transforming event for most people—or at least it appeared that it wasn't.

Not surprisingly, however, this is probably how you would have felt if you had the flu at age thirty-four, and, by way of example, your body created that first renegade cell that eventually morphed into the cancer you noticed at age fifty. The point is that when these seismic events occur, it is sometimes impossible to see their connection to anything downstream, let alone forecast their potential for transforming your life.

In a similar vein, the transistor, which is the basic building block of the semiconductor revolution, became the equivalent of a renegade cell for the computer industry. It provided the first in a series of building blocks that eventually led to where we are today: enjoying the power to create ever smaller and more powerful forms of processing and incorporate machine-based intelligence in our lives.

Is there a way to calculate or predict how a certain action or event that occurs today will transform our lives at some future, undetermined time? The goal of a system of PHC is to get us there, but, it will first require a number of infrastructure transformations including the growth of our personal data records, the creation of data standards, and a general rethinking about how we live our lives and work with our emerging health teams.

The 1986 explosion at the Chernobyl nuclear power station in the Ukraine represents an example of a destructive environmental force that would likely be included, for example, in a comprehensive health record of the various individuals exposed to the radioactive aftermath of the Chernobyl reactor. In the neighborhoods immediately surrounding Chernobyl, the causal relationship between X-rays and downstream illnesses were obvious. Victims suffered from dramatic exposures that caused nearly immediate changes to their cells with a resulting pattern of immediate illness.

But what about the vast majority of other cases—those in which the exposure rates were not as clear, or they were not as closely linked as was the Chernobyl community? These larger clusters of individuals exemplify the problems and opportunities of data mining and knowledge creation. Given the complexity of this biological-chemical problem, where do we find our answer?

The answer will eventually emerge through the growth of reference databases that contain an evolving collection of "known" relationships of data elements to physical outcomes.

Creating a reference database like the ones being used in the credit-scoring industry is relatively easy. The amount of information required to determine whether you continue paying your bills or can qualify for some type of loan to help you through the rough patch is fairly nominal. However, this is definitely not the case when you starting mixing organic (people) and inorganic (raw material such as chemicals) together and try to establish predictive relationships.

Remember when you began to appreciate the wonders of chemistry as a child? For the vast majority of us, our careers as amateur chemists demonstrated how little we understood of the actual causal relationships of compounds or mixtures of chemicals.

Transfer that limited knowledge base to the modern world and think of the incredible and expansive array of chemical and energy forces we subject our bodies to and you may begin to appreciate that we are all simply examples of living chemistry experiments. Since no master chemist is on hand as we purposely or accidentally create potentially horrific situations for our bodies, we have good reason to fear. It is these subtle relationships that will be so hard to uncover, yet even more important to understand as we move into our future systems of PHC.

The Internet has, in many ways, provided the missing piece of the puzzle to solving our crisis in the health care industry. And we have clearly excelled, as the chapters on data and data harvesting highlighted, in finding ever more clever ways of capturing information on our bodies.

The big question is now that we have the data—and the tools— what are we going to do with it? Google has at least provided us with a starting point and demonstrated how the Internet can be used to parse through an unlimited universe of information—and to expand and reconfigure its searching based on the dynamic and evolving content housed within the Internet's various nodes.

But as I hope you would appreciate, the answer to this question will impact all the "actors" of our health care system, including health professionals, the newly empowered patient, and the "churches" of health care, the hospital. Given the dynamic nature of relationships— and the complexity of dealing with humans—we should expect that building these future systems of connected information will not be easy. Creating a highway for cars is far easier than making sure that everyone follows the abstract standards facing our digital world.

At the end of the day it is easy to count cars on a highway. But how do you count and understand the digital bits that should be part of your future health record? And remember that dropping some "bits" of information off of that record is not a great idea—as our neighbors that lived around Chernobyl or Love Canal would attest. Knowing more is not a luxury; it is a requirement.

So who around us is either clever enough or has the collective smarts to tackle this problem? Dee Hock may be one of them.

CHAPTER 11

FACILITIES REDEFINED

THE YEAR 1968 was a banner one for the financial community. No, it was not a time that the stock market took off. The late 1990s was a period where irrational emotions demonstrated how to make and lose a ton of money through investments. But 1968 was not that time.

And no we did not have a stock market crash the way we did in 1929.

In 1968 an important and pervasive industry—*the business of credit cards*—redefined itself through the use of an innovative model of community. It started with a meeting in Columbus, Ohio, that I bet absolutely none of you knew was taking place—or have heard about since. But the results of that meeting have impacted almost everyone.

The agenda for the meeting was contentious: how to deal with the major financial problems taking place in the credit card industry. According to M. Waldrop from a 1996 article in *Fast Company*, "Children were getting cards. Pets were getting cards. Convicted felons were getting cards. Fraud was rampant, and the banks were hemorrhaging red ink."[1]

The credit card industry was a mess. Worse for the industry: there was no end in sight to this ongoing disaster. Enter the thinking of Dee Hock and at least one solution to the problem.

Hock is not a name that most people recognize. He built a business that even today most people would be hard pressed to figure out—VISA. Ask anyone where the VISA Company has its headquarters and their response will be a blank expression.

Why? Because VISA headquarters don't exist, at least not in the form we are accustomed to seeing as we drive (or hopefully walk) past the monolithic office towers in our modern urban centers.

Certainly VISA has a system of operations and control. But in developing its business, it required that the banking industry, and specifically credit cards, be built in a way that unified a diverse community of providers while at the same time allowing these providers to maintain their unique identity. The VISA philosophy was to provide basic tools, a network, and the rules of the road, and then let the competition work within an organized environment.

In the process of solving this banking nightmare, Hock had invented a new model of social organization he labeled Chaordic—the merger of chaotic and ordered approaches.

The delivery of health care has a number of issues similar to what Hock faced in 1968—local control that requires centralized thinking. The question is whether and how his Chaordic model can be utilized to redefine our health care system.

The Future Health Network

The health care economy is large. Consuming over $2 trillion annually (2006) of the U.S. GDP, it has grown into one of the world's largest employers through a complicated maze of institutions with little to no integration between the various parts of the "system.

First, there is absolutely no one in charge.

From the day you were born and for all your days thereafter, your interactions with the health care industry were, at best, random. You were neither provided with a maintenance roadmap for your body nor were you given a single point of contact for resolving issues. When you got ill or were injured, chances are you were left to your own devices to figure out where to go for care—with the landscape of providers constantly shifting. Moreover, you had no real sense for what health care cost until it was far too late in the process.

When was the last time you did price/value shopping in this market?

Good luck if you came down with a serious illness and were without medical insurance. If this were the case, and it happens to countless Americans every day, it is extremely likely you would have wound up financially destitute as the various "systems" of health care would have consumed absolutely every financial resource you had. The leading cause of personal bankruptcy is due to the costs of health care.

From the pharmaceutical industry, to the third-party payer community, to hospitals and physicians, the modern U.S. health care system represents one of the world's greatest examples of economic disincentives. Unfortunately, it has also become an incredibly large machine to feed.

By the early years of the twenty-first century, there were over 7,000 hospitals, more than 800,000 physicians and surgeons, and over 2.4 million nurses in the United States working on or contributing to the over 33 million inpatients (per year). And it came at a cost of over $500 billion.[2]

Can we expect more of the same growth in the coming era of PHC? Probably not and here's why. First on the list of reasons is the matter of where health care and medical treatment will occur in the future.

The modern hospital has evolved into a collection of care-delivery silos, with their needs sometimes interrelated but often existing in isolation. An emergency department, for example, is designed to provide immediate trauma care, so by its very definition, it must contend with whatever shows up in its door. In contrast, a surgical suite often services the scheduled needs of patients and cases and has a reasonable idea on when its "customers" will arrive.

Any discussion of the future PHC-driven hospital must begin with a focus on these atomic units. Because although a hospital is often viewed as part of a system, the reality is that it operates through a variety of clinical programs supported by administrative infrastructures. And while we may not like to believe it, the modern hospital has more in common with your traditional shopping center that you would probably like to hear. It definitely does not work like the more modern automobile manufacturing plants of Toyota or the semiconductor facilities of Intel.

So, where we do start? One of the areas in which we can expect to find numerous innovations—and will continue to be a critical component of our future system—is the operating room (OR). It is also starting to embrace the various technical revolutions underpinning our movement to PHC.

New Surgical Suite

Several key factors governing the design of a hospital's OR will more than likely be similar in the future world of PHC. You can be confident, for example, that your hospital will maintain a focus on ensuring that the OR environment and atmosphere are clean, appropriate sterile equipment is being used, properly trained personnel are manning the ship, and life-support systems are readily available to help keep you alive during the procedure.

Technology will drive a number of modern updates, including the use of sensor technologies to alert the health team when things have gone awry. Data points, it turns out, can come from a wide variety of places, with the OR being one of the many that we will be adding to the expansive repositories of health information.

Another interesting element of the future OR will be the likely increased use of real-time navigation systems to aid the surgical team. You should expect to find another set of eyes and hands driven by information known and obtained during the procedure peering over you as you lie on the operating table. You should also expect to find an increased use of intraoperative imaging and robotic surgery tools. These additional tools are examples of machine-based intelligence I discussed earlier and highlighted by the work of Dr. Russell Taylor in his research.

Along with the use of these machine utilities, we can expect to see the addition of a new family of data-driven interventions requiring even more granularity taken from our human maps. People are decidedly not all the same, and a new generation of human maps will be required to provide a personalized connection to the targeted therapies that are already evolving through lasers, focused ultrasound, and gamma knives.

Who will lead the OR team?

My assumption is that the actual procedures performed within an OR will continue under some form of human leadership. Will that leader still be a master surgeon or some other member of the health professional team? And will the surgeon or health professionals guiding the procedure remain physically located within the OR?

In the end, the actual leader of the future surgical pack will more than likely come from a mix of players. It is my guess that in complex medical situations, requiring highly specialized knowledge and problem-solving skills gained through years of rigorous training, an expert surgeon would lead the team. In the wider array of other more predictable cases, and especially those that can rely on a closely monitored integration of information-guided technologies and real-time feedback, my guess is that a newer class of less skilled professionals will head the charge, although with access to an emerging virtual world of supporters.

One of the great innovations of the Internet has been the ability to coalesce expertise across disciplines and from distinct geographic regions of the world. Where proximity was at one time the only reliable way of gleaning feedback from your colleagues, the future OR will likely include the ability to directly link experts within a dynamic electronic community. Get confused during the procedure and these newer community devices will allow you to immediately extend your own knowledge base and include the thinking of other distant professionals in your procedures.

Why, for example, would you not want to have the input of an expert surgeon from Denver assisting your local team in Dayton? The answer is that you would and for a variety of reasons including better outcomes.

The supporting players driving this future OR will include an expanding collection of technologies, spanning wireless communications and "smart dust" sensors to live information feeds similar to those used on Wall Street. Given the advances in decision-support applications, we can also assume that a variety of "intelligent" programs (similar to the Internist application I described earlier) will monitor the health of the patient and the course of the procedure to ensure everything is proceeding as planned. Finally, control process systems will be in place to assure proper management of the information relevant to the procedure, and feedback loops will drive equipment-controlling systems as fundamental as anesthesiology and life support.

Now let's shift from the operating theater to the intensive care units (ICU)—the place in a hospital for those with life-threatening consequences of disease and trauma or recovering from a recent operation.

Intensive Care Units

An ICU represents the single most complex environment of a hospital. It contains some of the facility's most sophisticated technologies, often housing patients in the last stages of their lives—with their survival measured on a moment-to-moment basis. While an OR is complicated and involves a number of potentially lethal interactions, the future ICU will be required as the life support of last resort, offering the patient the types of mechanical and chemical assistance their bodies simply cannot provide any longer. It is in this complex environment that some of the more impressive life-altering impacts of PHC will be felt.

Relying on the growing knowledge of the individual's human map and integrating a number of the evolving reference databases, the future ICU will deal with each patient through a highly personalized set of management approaches. Knowing how an entire population responds bears little importance when you are dealing with an individual whose life status can change any second. The ICU is thus one of the best places to discard the concept of averages.

The ideal treatment for a dying patient should be tuned to the patient's unique definition of average response, which will more than likely include some combination of knowledge of their genome, environment, and what we have gained over time through a more detailed analysis of their life equation and the now millions of data points obtained over time and housed within their personal health record. Yes, science and medicine have entered an era of intense usage of data and analytics.

If, for example, we understand the ways in which a patient's body responds to tissue regeneration, its care delivery team can create more highly tuned and efficient treatment programs that recognize this difference.

Assuming we continue to experience the impacts of Gordon Moore's Law (i.e., the statement by Moore that "the number of transistors and resistors on a chip doubles every 18 months"[3]), we should also anticipate further miniaturizations in the size of the ICU's equipment, along with reductions in cost and dramatic increases in their native intelligence. Just as the EKG has morphed into a smart box with a footprint that can fit in your hand, a wide array of new smart monitoring applications should replace the current array of big machines and complicated interfaces.

When you turn the key in the ignition of your car you begin a carefully orchestrated series of interactions, all governed by a complex array of sensors and switches. Why not have the same types of interactions with the complex machinery and feedback loops within these future ICUs?

As the movement to machine intelligence has demonstrated, and the work of Dr. Lee Goldman in Chicago emphasized, the use of carefully constructed algorithms can improve patient outcomes. The future ICU will include this type of thinking in absolutely every system it uses to support the patients its serves.

Moving beyond the surgical faculties and the machine-intensive support systems required within ICUs, the remaining silos of the hospital are also likely to undergo a dramatic restructuring. For an example of these changes, let's look first at the specialized discipline of oncology. Will hospitals be the place you go for cancer therapies?

The Emerging Model of Disease Treatment

One of the more critical areas of medical treatment for our health care system is in managing the disease stages of cancer. The expansive range of this disease requires a number of treatment programs that often bring the patient to a hospital—establishing an interesting set of parallels with other illnesses that also require hospital encounters.

Our future cases of a cancer treatment program may still require surgery, and the interactions with the hospital will likely continue to mirror other surgical procedures. However, remember a key point: in the ultimate system of PHC, our objective will be to have identified and managed that growing cancer long before it required surgery. For those cases that require surgery you can expect the last thing anyone will do is physically cut a patient open. The amount of innovation and R&D focused on noninvasive methods of diagnosis and treatment is staggering, with the real potential to view inpatient cancer treatments as more complex ambulatory visits. Yes, you will probably be required to visit a hospital-style facility for your treatments. But once there you will sustain less physical damage through a combination of targeted therapies and advanced pharmaceuticals serving as the modern scalpel.

What will be the driver of these cases and what will be used to establish the most appropriate treatment approach? Again, information and the human map will serve as the platform for both discovery and treatment.

What about those cases that cannot be solved by a future surgical approach and require some type of medical treatment? It is here that you will begin to see the dramatic and immediate value of our movement to PHC.

Today's chemotherapies flood the body with toxic chemicals that preferentially destroy fast-growing cells—including cancer cells, but also, unfortunately, other cells we'd like to keep, like hair. In our evolving therapies of PHC, the old type of chemotherapy will be supplanted by a series of targeted medications that leave almost everything else in your body intact—with only the cancerous cells being the ones with something to worry about. The resulting impact is that your body is generally happier and you, the patient, will suffer from fewer nasty side effects while accelerating your recovery time.

The underlying theme in both the medical and surgical treatments of our systems of PHC is information—and how it is compared to existing knowledge, mapped back to the patient, and then used as the planning tool for the plan of attack. Where will all of this diagnostic data (labs and radiology) be generated that defines our new health care system? The answer is everywhere.

Omnipresent Diagnostics

As I hope you have now come to appreciate, the evolution of PHC and its impact on medical treatments will require information on you, the patient, that can be easily accessed and in some cases brought along with you to shape your treatment plan. So where will this information be coming from?

Although the discussion on reference databases highlights just how complex this information-gathering task will be, requiring us to obtain from nontraditional sources and to have that information included in our personal health record, the vast majority of your traditional data points will be coming from the data-harvesting programs I introduced earlier. But you are lucky on this front. The advent and growth of the modern diagnostic approaches (X-ray through PCR) represent a few of the seminal events that occurred in the twentieth century—and they are about to become almost transparent.

You can expect that in our future systems of PHC, diagnostics will move everywhere and in many ways parallel the migration of computer technology as it slowly becomes a ubiquitous part of our world.

The concept of having to travel to a hospital or clinic to understand your body chemistry, for example, will more than likely be replaced by a collection of home-based technologies allowing you to perform real-time assessments with the results immediately embedded within your personal health record. These results will also be automatically routed to the professionals who are part of your team and subjected to an array of decision-support routines. They, in turn, will provide you with feedback that may be used to adjust your living patterns or to seek some additional help.

What will enable this data-to-action cycle? Simple, it will be the NHIN (or its equivalent local model) and a variety of computer applications. Remember how the EKG evolved from requiring operator analysis to having the machine doing the work?

For more complex diagnostic tests you may have to drive to your corner drug store or self-service diagnostic center, which will provide full service access to a wide array of the more complicated diagnostic measures—including those requiring the use of chemical markers and other technical approaches to evaluate the mechanical and chemical aspects of your body's functions that you simply cannot do in a "portable" environment.

Now that you have all of this data and your populated human map, where do you think you will be receiving your everyday health care services? One answer is that it may be coming from your drugstore.

Retail Health Services

The CVS Corporation has been leading a revolution in thinking about health care services. In 2006, it acquired a company, Minute Clinics, that had introduced a novel idea to the health care community—freestanding triage centers focused on the easy-to-manage health problems and assessments embedded within a traditional retail center. If you think you have the flu, stop into this 300 to 400 square-foot facility and you will get an immediate answer, and at a cost you can afford or, at a minimum, understand.

With Minute Clinic you can forget the confusion of insurance—what is the price of what I am paying for anyway? And you can forget the waiting room and the dehumanizing clutter of the traditional physician practice. How many people would say that going to their doctor's office is a pleasant experience or that the staff in their doctor's office treated them the same way the sales person from Nordstrom's did? The answer is close to zero.

Minute Clinic was thinking retail and understood that their customers wanted easy and fast service. Their small clinics, which by the end of 2006 were now being housed within CVS drugstores, were the answer to at least part of the access problem (and pent-up demand) in health care and a sign of what the future of our front-end systems will look like.

No, the doctor's office is not being replaced. I doubt that anyone involved in this new retail health care industry believes that the Minute Clinic model will solve the current crisis on the primary care end of our health care system. But I do believe it represents a sign of the times and a wakeup call for the rest of the industry. Patients are, in the end, consumers and will be demanding prices that they can understand, high quality service, and, finally, convenience.

I also suggest that retail health care (like Minute Clinic) is the beginning of the shift to a system of PHC, with its requirement for flexible delivery environments and easy patient access. Remember that the model for PHC demands information and that patients have the ability to easily act on it. Minute Clinic, if nothing else, provides one example of how to provide that service.

The impact of all of these changes will be our shift in orientation away from thinking of the physical plant of health care as being the hospital, and replaced by an array of treatment programs, facilities, and technical support. Telehealth and the emerging machine-based applications described by the VisiCu team only add fuel to this transformational fire.

The hospital may have been the sacred ground of health care in the past, but its days are numbered. But where will doctors fit in this new world?

Notes

1. M. Waldrop, "The Trillion-Dollar Vision of Dee Hock," *Fast Company* Issue 5 (October 1996): 75.

2. U.S. Census Bureau, April 2005.

3. G. Moore, "Cramming More Components onto Integrated Circuits," *Electronics* 38, no. 8 (April 19, 1965).

CHAPTER 12

THE NEW PROFESSIONALS AND PATIENTS

MEDICINE IS ONE of the world's oldest and most respected professions. It comes with a tremendous social and psychological responsibility, as the medical professional is often faced with the devastating impacts of illness and disease suffered by their patients and the need to guide them through their health journey. Our emerging systems of personalized health care (PHC) are about to transform the roles of this noble profession as its redefines the patient's health team.

Figure 12.1 provides some insight into the newer collection of health care professionals our reconstructed system of health care will require. Some you recognize, others may seem strange. Yet the largest component of change in this figure is something that may not be obvious—the theme of "systems" and "team."

How will this change the relationships of the various "actors" of our health care community—including patients, professionals, and health facilities? First will be in reshaping who manages your health journey and experiences.

The Coach as the Practice

Imagine what it would be like to play basketball without a coach. On the one hand, it could be viewed as the ultimate freedom. You practice with your teammates, play your schedule while hopefully winning games, and keeping your grades up. You may get good enough,

Figure 12.1. 19th- versus 21st-Century Care Providers

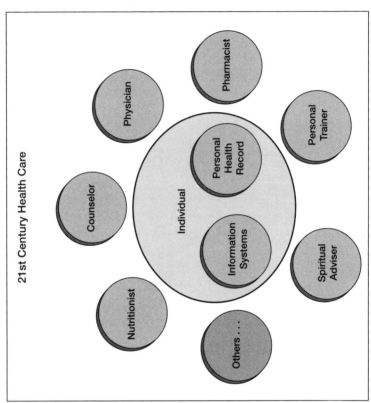

on your own to make it to the pros. You have the ability to create and achieve individually, based solely on your own individual skills.

The problem with this model is that it never happens. One of the things we have learned, as a general rule, is that without some form of mentoring, it is tough to improve and make the best use of your innate talents and skills. Coaches typically offer a broad base of knowledge and experience, and more than likely can push your development beyond what you could have accomplished on your own.

The same is true with how you manage your health. In the past, we had a health coach we could turn to for help—the family doctor. Doctors might not have been able to solve all of our health problems, but they were there with emotional support and ideas that often made it easier to overcome our immediate health woes. With the advent of the scientific practice of medicine, handholding disappeared and society shifted its focus to diseases and how to manage them.

The holistic approaches of the past were ushered out as we created a system with multiple providers, each having access to specific expertise, along with a new arsenal of treatments. Given the number of technical changes taking place in the field of medicine, it was an evolution that made sense and was probably the only way of applying the flood of new knowledge to patient care.

The explosive growth of data mining and support models of the information age gives us the opportunity to rethink our current manner of delivering health care, and in doing so, brings back the coaches to help us navigate the health questions we face throughout life.

On one hand, we have questions about how to optimize our health status. How do we ensure we are tuning the machine in the best way we possibly can? On the other hand, we wonder what to do when things go wrong. What are the best options? How should I decide what to do? Going it alone is not the best answer for most of us, nor are we likely to get the best answers solely from our physician.

Clearly, experiments in alternative health and coaching are already taking place. But the rise of alternative medicine can, on one level, be seen as a reaction by the patient marketplace to the lack of coaching and individualized care the consumer craves. We are faced with complex issues and not having the relationship of the past (i.e., the nineteenth-century handholding), we look for help wherever we can get it.

What does the future hold? A good bet is that the ultimate system of PHC will eventually include an ever-changing team of professionals, with the physician-patient relationship still a major component.

The foundation of this new practice architecture is the health/life model discussed earlier, its interaction with your life equation and the support of the care delivery team that helps you manage specific elements of your health/disease journey. Connected to this delivery and support architectures will be the wide array of data points that will be generated around you and housed within personal health records that serve as the communication engine for your now virtual health care system.

The important point is that your future systems of health care—and the way in which you interact with its various system components—will be focused on three basic elements: you, your health team, and your data encounters. And no, it will not simply be one of the old symbols of the health care industry: the hospital and the doctor.

Yes, these historic symbols of the past will still be important and relevant. But they will not be the entire story and they will also not be the defining architecture. The management of health will follow a continuum, with convergences of virtual and physical facilities and programs—and a renewed sense of community.

Technology will not, by itself, lead the migration of our health system into the new age of the knowledge economy. Ultimately, the new system of PHC will represent a convergence of technological, social, and economic forces. It will also usher in an era in which we measure the quality of life by how well we can maintain optimal health. And we will have a number of twenty-first-century tools and providers to make sure we get there.

Are these new tools an example of a "facility" or a "professional?" I am not sure how to classify them since they contain a mixture of both and build upon almost every element of the technologies driving our movement to PHC.

Moving to Virtual

The Internet has permanently changed the control and distribution of knowledge and altered every aspect of how we obtain and use information in our lives. Consider how it could influence the most fundamental of all of the exchanges—the question of an illness and the visit to a physician.

Would you want to spend the time scheduling an appointment, waiting days or weeks, driving to the doctor's office, and then waiting to see your physician when you could get a quick response over the Internet in the privacy of your home or office?

According to the National Ambulatory Medical Care Survey, Americans made approximately 910 million office visits to their physicians in the year 2004. Factoring in travel time and a waiting factor along with the actual visit (let's conservatively say a total of three hours), these 910 million visits added up to over 2.7 billion hours of time, which equates to 113 million days or 311,000 years. Considering that the average life span of someone living in the United States is only seventy-seven years, a whole lot of productivity is lost due to those hours upon hours of waiting.[1] We are consuming the equivalent of over 40,000 people's lives each year simply driving to physicians' offices, waiting in their lobby, and getting their advice and counsel. There has got to be a better way of delivering this service.

When we discussed the activities of Drs. Mike Breslow and Brian Rosenfeld they were focused on the challenges of monitoring patients in an ICU. Breslow and Rosenfeld felt that the current use of a wandering doctor on the floor was not the most efficient solution and eventually constructed an information-based alternative housing remote monitoring program and a "command and control" system.

The Breslow/Rosenfeld point was basic: why not optimize the abilities and time of the physician through an elegant model of decision-support applications and sensor-based data acquisition?

Merge Breslow and Rosenfeld's work with that of Dr. Dadong Wan on the Magic Medicine Cabinet and you get an idea of how this new world will work and can be applied to most doctor-patient interchanges, and not just in the ICU.

The utility of a combined Breslow/Rosenfeld/Wan model is almost limitless. Assume you have some knowledgeable individual on one end of the communications pipeline and the appropriate level of sensor-based information coming from the other—the basic telehealth architecture. Telehealth solutions promise the potential to dramatically extend the reach of the health care system and help physicians as well as patients recoup the time wasted in the archaic system of "land-based" information exchanges, while at the same time introducing the concepts of real-time management of health. It is a set of solutions that is already beginning to hit the marketplace.

Imagine a world where you can follow the health activities of a sick parent or relative a thousand miles away through a sensor and biometric-driven information network, just like their personal health care provider manually does today and in person. The electronic community model of CTSNet and its extensions provides an elegant and robust platform for defining new ways of staying in touch—far beyond the simple exchange of a telephone call—and are additional examples of the potential of technology to transform.

From the challenges of consulting on a faraway patient to managing the medical conditions of a local patient with congestive heart failure, telehealth solutions will no doubt become one of the platform elements of the newly configured system of PHC, with a visit to the doctor (or other member of your health team) no longer defined by your driving to their office. This convergence of technologies will also reintroduce the historical concept of physicians making house calls, albeit through a very different model of how they interact. E-mail, telehealth, and the Internet will become extremely valuable partners in the process of managing your health.

The vast innovations defined in the twentieth century created distance between both patients and their health status and patients and their health providers. However, in the twenty-first century, technology will help correct this imbalance as it becomes the new foundation for the practices of PHC. Restating the paradox of the opening chapter, as an interesting twist of fate, technology will be used to rehumanize our health care system.

Navigating the Future Health System

How will the move to personalization impact the broader health care system of patients, providers, employers, and payers? Most of the convergence to PHC will be powered by fundamental solutions in knowledge management. As most of us will come to appreciate, the physician-patient relationship will evolve to include a broader team of players, preventive action, and the recognition that each individual contains a wealth of complex and unique genetic roadmaps. The gene was a starting point that, when combined with the way the individual lived his life, determined his health status. But it is not enough.

In the knowledge era, the system of health care will no longer be defined by physical infrastructure, such as the hospitals, clinics, and doctors who had come to define health care in the past. With the help of your health coach, doctor, and the rest of your personal health "team," your ability to manage your health will in large part rest with your understanding of your own unique set of biological markers and how you utilize that information to maintain your health and prevent disease.

No longer viewed as a series of isolated events, these markers will come to signify your health status—and will provide early clues when your body is beginning to have problems. Call it prospective or preventative, the objective is the same—to control and influence a later-stage health outcome. And unlike playing the roulette wheel, maintaining health is not simply a matter of chance. It's a game of probability and relative risks.

So assume that in working with your team, you agree that it is time for the next round of checkups, based on a microarray analysis indicating you have one or two questionable genes, along with a family history of breast cancer. You then enter a process of guided assessment that will more than likely involve the work of specialized diagnostic equipment and the support of technologists and physicians. With the results in hand—and in this case I will assume you have now been diagnosed with an early stage breast cancer, for example—you return with the results of a biopsy for a discussion with your doctor/ coach about a best-fit treatment.

You, along with the increasing number of health professionals on your care management team, will begin exploring the options that may be best for you. These possibilities might be based on the fact that the particular signature of your cancer, combined with your genetics, makes you an ideal candidate for a new drug targeted to your unique combination of disease and physiology. Along with the use of this innovative new product of the pharmacogenomics revolution and the decision support provided by your health team's knowledge repository, you may decide that your best predicted outcome would be to surgically remove the early stage tumor. How will you find the most appropriate facility to perform the surgery?

Again, with the help of your team and the resources of your health information system, you will select a facility with an outstanding track record in performing the specific type of surgical procedure you require based on an analysis of the various performance metrics of that facility. Such an analysis includes various measures of surgical outcomes, customer satisfaction, and costs.

Working again with your team, you will enter the surgical facility and have the tumor removed—all within the schedule you have outlined and with appropriate levels of support throughout. The results of the postsurgical examination of the tumor are immediately communicated to your team and included in your now-expanding personal health record.

After leaving the treatment facility, you will return to a discussion with your health coach and determine—based on the data acquired during and after your surgery—that the specific cancer you have is an ideal fit for a pharmacogenomic treatment program slightly different than the one identified at the time of the original diagnosis.

Your postsurgical treatment is again based on actions you determine with the support of knowledge from your health information analysis. Here you are confronted with a number of options. On one hand, you could improve your potential survival rate by electing to use a hard-hitting combination of therapies with the downside being that this would potentially reduce your quality of life. The alternative pathway would reduce the likelihood of a cure but would also lessen the risk of negative side effects. With advice from your personal health care team, and the virtual community of cancer patients (and their families) receiving both treatment options, you will decide which course is best for you. The treatment begins, seems to work as anticipated, you continue your follow-ups with your team with your health coach leading the way.

What is wrong with this scenario? Clearly the goal of the future systems of PHC would be to have helped you avoid getting the cancer in the first place. Had we all of the information, knowledge of all of the compounding relationships, and acted accordingly you—the patient in this example—would never have shown up with breast cancer. Forgetting this ultimate objective for a moment (i.e., avoiding the cancer rather than having to treat it), a fascinating element of this story is that it did not once mention the word "hospital" or "specialized facility." The many elements of your discovery and action path were almost exclusively centered on the challenges of data management—with information acquired through your personal health record as well as from analysis using the provider's information warehouse. How this information was discussed within the health team and how they engaged the treatment pathways of the health care delivery system were the key components of your decision support.

Now get ready for the big change, the rise of the empowered patient. You are, for the first time in your health care life, about to be put in charge.

The Empowered Patient

What does the future hold for us as health care consumers? The starting point will be a reorientation, with one of the most critical being a recognition that our lives are filled with a series of action/reactions unfolding over time and that we are moving through life facing a series of choices and exposures that will have an impact on our future health and quality of life. As we discussed earlier, we are not always sure where and when they will appear—or where they will lead. Our life equation is complicated, with the possible variations of our human map and our actions conspiring to define an almost infinite number of possibilities.

Nonetheless we must understand that there is a relationship between action and reaction, no matter how abstract or how far away. Figure 12.2 highlights this new orientation, in which you begin to recognize the various decision-impact points in your life—and that they could shorten your time on earth, or reduce your ability to enjoy the time you have.

Unfortunately, the transformation from immediate to long-term thinking will be difficult. Would the citizens of Love Canal, for example, have stayed in their houses had they understood the noxious odor of their neighborhoods was slowly changing the internal

Figure 12.2. Life Path and Choices

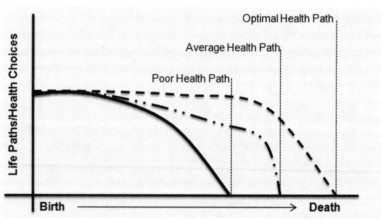

scripts of their life equation? We wake each morning and generally live through a series of one-at-a-time responses. Some of these actions are purely motor driven and controlled by our brains as our body adjusts to its environment. You take for granted, for example, that your body can easily balance as it moves through space. Placing one foot in front of another and walking requires little control by you, other than the conscious decision to move. The brain takes care of all of the subtle adjustments required by your muscles to ensure you don't topple over.

But how often do you think beyond the moment—and how your actions will influence your long-term health? For most of us, the answer is not much at all, with school being one of the few places that forces us to think about the future.

Consider the time when you entered first grade. The traditional systems of education represent a classic example of forward and future thinking. Each successive school year builds upon your successes from the prior years while your knowledge grows incrementally. It is society's method of maturation along with an easy-to-understand path of moving from one stage of life to another.

Living forward is the broad concept of recognizing that your actions will lead to some downstream series of rewards or goals. For school, this could represent new career opportunities, wealth, and social standing. You are acting with the knowledge that your actions can have the potential to influence your outcome—and what you are able to achieve and realize. As anyone in retail industries understands, living forward is one of the most critical relationships needed to understand where to locate a store and decide which products to place on its shelves. Retailers like Wal-Mart make this a science.

Unfortunately for those of us who are worried about the health care system, the thinking-forward model rarely applies to how individuals deal with their bodies. When we think of health care issues, we often move away from the future action/reaction mode to more of a series of "one day at a time" events.

While recognizing the ultimate answer to this question is really a series of complex relationships between your own mental state and life's choices—and unfortunately often the result of either your own good or bad luck in where you genetically landed—we are presented with an often confusing set of alternatives with no clear idea of whether these options are valid and what their downstream benefits will include.

When I reviewed the mechanical construct and the concept of errors, one of the issues I did not discuss was life span. Clearly, almost all of us deal with this thinking when we move through our lives. We understand, for example, that the number of miles we can put on our cars is finite. There aren't too many of us driving around in vehicles with 3 million miles on them.

Cars, like almost all mechanical devices, have a life span. Eventually, they stop working. Yes, in the case of a car, one could argue that almost all of the pieces could be replaced so, in effect, you would during the course of driving those 3 million miles have rebuilt the entire car through several mechanical lifetimes. But humans do not share that same luxury or option, at least given today's technical limitations.

This issue of informed and rational selection is one of the penultimate problems for the emerging systems of PHC. We can easily think of a retirement account and saving for the future. We can move through school and gain the right skills for that projected dream job. Yet, for some reason, we have been unable to generally apply that same long-term thinking to our health. Given the vast number of mixed messages we receive from society and how confusing the mechanics/missions of living really are, is there any way of thinking forward in health care?

Maybe. And here is one way of starting the process.

Note

1. Centers for Disease Control, "National Ambulatory Care Medical Survey: 2004 Summary," June 2006.

CONCLUSION
An Industry in Motion

S
TEVEN JOBS did not invent the radio. He also did not invent recorded music.

And, as everyone involved with the growth of the transistor, the semiconductor, the microprocessor, and the eventual personal computer will note, he did not create the computer industry, either.

But he did reinvent Apple and did so in a way that almost no one would have predicted. He intuitively recognized the convergence of digital media and the memories that music brings each time you rehear a song, and by doing so, he rebuilt the revolution of the transistor radio.

> Whenever Jason Berkowitz listens to "You're the Best" on his iPod, he recalls that 1984 summer vacation in Fort Lauderdale and seeing *The Karate Kid* for the first time. ("I thought it was the best song ever. I still kinda do and I don't care what people say," says the 29-year-old). Whenever he listens to Zero 7's song "Destiny," which he first heard at London's Heathrow Airport four years ago, he thinks about meeting his wife, Bethany.[1]

The short history of the iPod reflects everything Steven Jobs does well. Packaging, function, branding, and market rollouts have become legend—and a model for how to innovate within the computer industry. But what Jobs accomplished with the iPod is a great example of something else—the power to reinvent a seemingly intransigent industry.

Changing how health care is delivered to our bedside, at home, and for our parents and friends will require a similar set of new ideas and thinking. It also will enjoy the advantages that almost all elements of the system stand to gain—and are looking for something new. It is a set of changes that the health care industry has seen in the past. The business of medicine and health has been tested by new knowledge and the need for new models many times before. The professional growth of physicians, the rise of complex tertiary care centers, and the evolving basic sciences all represent the inherent push of the industry to innovate. The movement to a personal view of health is, in many ways, simply the next chapter of the history of this noble science.

Until recently, most Americans had little idea of the costs of their health care. It was an invisible system of benefits in which employers managed the employee's health. The agent that most of us came to know was an amorphous organization known as the managed-care company that would establish contracts with physicians, health networks, and others involved in the delivery and support of the health care system—including pharmaceuticals.

And until the late twentieth century, almost no one really cared about this collection of support players because, quite frankly, none of us were put in the position where we had to think about it, let alone take control of it. For most employees, health was a benefit and an entitlement we took for granted. Managing our health was generally mysterious to us and left to the control of experts.

The system started showing cracks in its foundation when the reality of its economic model demonstrated its weakness—and the costs of care became unacceptable, even to corporations that basically accepted health costs as a part of doing business. The unfortunate reality is that our health care economy was built with no effective system of checks and balances, leaving the economic players free to inflate and charge in whatever way that made sense to them but not necessarily to those who paid the bill—employees, employers, and tax payers.

When this reality became apparent to each of those groups, the status quo was no longer acceptable. The train wreck of escalating costs began to hit and did so with a vengeance.

So how did the system react? The first response was a move to squeeze costs on the providers of care, with the first to feel the crunch being the provider system: the physicians and hospitals. The next change to the system was even more interesting—raising the price to the customer. How? By keeping monthly benefits of employees the same but forcing them to start picking up some or all of the costs.

The final movement, which has already begun, is rationing. Unfortunately, rationing is a bad approach without a system of replacements and a market-driven economy of informed choices. But it is an easy solution in times of crisis and poor planning.

The net is that we have tried to adjust the pricing models, reduce reimbursement, and change payers, but none of these traditional tools have worked. We ended the twentieth century by trimming the costs of the suppliers—the employees of the health system—and began the twenty-first century by raising the price to customers. But if the revolutions of personalized health care (PHC) take hold, our future systems will have shifted to rational market pricing and accurate market information. How will this happen?

The answer is through the convergence of economic interests of the government, employers, and patients and the laws of supply and demand. We are living within a global and connected economy in which the costs of doing business will move to equilibriums. The U.S. health care system represents one of the world's great imbalances, with every employer and our government facing severe competitive issues moving forward. The migration to a new way of thinking about health is rapidly becoming less an option and more a requirement—we can no longer afford to provide health care coverage the old way.

What will be the future metrics that will be replacements to the traditional models of price and volume that the industry thinks about today? These will be replaced by a metric that any good retailer understands, namely outcomes, cost, and customer satisfaction. We are heading to a consumer-driven economic model of health care governed by rationale market forces.

In the perfect world of health care, each of the patient/consumer's market activities will be based on information and knowledge of alternatives and consequences. Our future systems of PHC have the potential to provide that information and more. The system, thanks to a number of converging forces, is starting to change. Get ready to meet the empowered and healthy patient.

"Doctor, the patient is ready to see you now."[2]

Return to the Beginning

In closing I would like to revisit the opening challenge of the book and the question of what will be required to "fix" our current health care system: is universal health insurance, for example, the answer to our current health crisis? Do we need to build more hospitals or educate more physicians?

I hope that by now you can answer these questions and appreciate that the deeper issue is how well you know your body, its potential, and the relationship of your actions to your health status. Providing insurance may be good for building economic incentives, but it lacks the depth of analysis and thinking that our health care system deserves—and that Sir William Osler would have recommended were he alive today.

So what do I believe is the answer to our current health care crisis? To me the answer is the basic but elegant function of $H = f(A, G, E)$ I described earlier. Imagine the world we would have if we were able to discover the answers to this simple collection of variables? In the future world of PHC we should have the ability to at least start to understand their depth and meaning. Our rising technology revolution, the growth of personalized data warehouses, and our emerging new health team will provide us with a different set of support—and information that describes who we are, where we are living, and how our actions can influence our future.

It could be an exciting time—assuming we figure out how to take advantage of the inherent potential that each of us has—because the double-edged sword of the coming genomic revolution is that our bodies genetic potential can be used either as a vehicle for discrimination or as the ultimate testimony on the skills that are housed within our bodies.

Will this more positive outcome happen in the future? We had better hope that the present is no foreshadowing for this later period in our evolution. If history is the judge of the future, then the story down the road may not always be a good one.

Every time I drive by a homeless person or the public-housing projects in Baltimore I get just a bit sadder knowing that we may have missed finding the cure for cancer today—or composing a symphony equivalent to the great works of Beethoven—by not giving each member of our society the chance to use his or her unique and amazing talents. Wasting human potential is the greatest crime of a society.

And yes, we have figured out how to do that *really* well.

Notes

1. Jose Antonio Vargas, "The iPod: A Love Story Between Man, Machine," *Washington Post*, August 17, 2005.

2. A variation on the recent BUPA (British United Provident Association) ad campaign, "The Patient will see you now, doctor."

INDEX

ABOUT THE AUTHOR

CAREY JAMES KRIZ is the executive director of the American Academy of Urgent Care Medicine and the founder and CEO of the Prospective Health Corporation. Mr. Kriz's career path has taken him through stints at IBM (starting as a programmer in the early 1980s), to the Johns Hopkins School of Medicine (as a faculty member in radiology and a member of the Johns Hopkins Medicine executive committee), and a variety of startups. His activities have and continue to span the United States, Asia, and the GCC.